Life Interrupted

Visit www.booksurge.com to order additional copies.

CHRIS
M. TATEVOSIAN

LIFE
INTERRUPTED

2007

Life Interrupted

TABLE OF CONTENTS

Helping you to identify and eliminate the growth of the relationship-destroying "poor me" attitude that frequently accompanies chronic illness.

DEDICATION

For The Awesome Love We Once Shared, I Dedicate This To My Ex-wife, Rachel, And My Remarkable Stepson, Jesse. You Are In My Thoughts And Prayers Always.

And A Special Dedication To My Brothers, Knoop, Charlie, And Squatch, Without Whom Many Of My Most Incredible Memories And Life Experiences Would Have Never Taken Place, Because They Would Have Been Physically, Mentally, And Emotionally Impossible Or Maybe The Thoughts Would Not Have Even Crossed My Unaltered State Of Mind. Thank You, Guys. You're The Best.

INTRODUCTION:

L ife Interrupted—It's Not All About Me" is my story about dealing with how I unknowingly let my battle with the effects of multiple sclerosis destroy the most important, significant, loving, and incredibly caring relationship: a marriage steeped in so much love that no one could have predicted or imagined its demise. My experiences will illustrate to you the sneaky and destructive ways that the "Poor Me Attitude" will inevitably destroy the strongest loving relationship whether you intentionally or unintentionally avoid addressing the "situation." You need to hear this true, firsthand account of my life with multiple sclerosis, a chronic progressive disease, so that you can recognize and possibly stop your relationship-destroying "Poor Me Attitude" actions. It may be easy to interpret this book as a book of "don'ts" rather than a book of "do's". It is not my intention to tell you what to do or not do. Nor is my intention to tell you how to act or not act. Simply, I want to share with you my experiences with multiple sclerosis and what I have learned from these experiences. My hope is that you draw from them, identify similarities and avoid making the same relationship destroying mistakes.

By sharing my story with you, I'm hoping that my mistakes and negative behaviors function as warning signs. In other words, when you read my story, perhaps you will identify with the same behavior and want to stop this behavior so that your relationships are not destroyed. This is not a reprimand, rather an opportunity to slow things down and reflect on your situation. I hope my story provides an opportunity for you, perhaps, to become more aware of your own actions and behaviors, an opportunity to rethink your next actions. I have learned that mindfulness and reflection can reduce, if not eliminate completely, one's anger and anxiety. By reading my story and hearing my words, I ideally hope that your struggles ease and life becomes more of a joy.

For the longest time I was not sure if the need to share my story really existed; confirmation came to me in the most unlikely manner one evening. Who would have expected a phone call from a telemarketer to have been that confirming factor, but it was. I always believed that there were people suffering, living and experiencing similar situations as mine, but I could have never imagined the numbers. Nor could I have ever imagined the incredible need to let others know that they were not alone, and that they too could face and overcome this situation.

The other night, Beverly, a telemarketer, called and somehow during the course of her sales pitch we got into a conversation about the fact that I was writing a book, a self-help memoir, so to speak. I remember thinking if she felt she could interrupt my evening with her agenda, it was only fair that she let me do the same to her. Anyone who knows me knows that I am not a shy, self-inhibited individual. Just the opposite; I'm always looking for the opportunity to step into the limelight and where possible interject a little humor and charm. After telling her about the topic, she told me that she had colitis and that she and her husband were dealing with a lot of the same issues that I was addressing in my book, "Life Interrupted—It's Not All About Me."

Beverly asked what she could do to help her relationship and to stop her "Poor Me Attitude" from growing and destroying her relationship. It seemed that both she and her husband were so very frustrated and angry all the time. Her husband, who was aware of her illness, did not recognize or understand that both she and he needed to adjust to manage living their lives with her illness. For example, no matter how many times she explained to her husband that she needed a bathroom close by whenever they went out, he never seemed to recognize the need and legitimacy of her request. Even if he did, his aggravation and lack of compassion was blatantly evident.

Her husband would get upset and start an argument whenever she expressed her concern regarding the location, accessibility, and conveniences of the restroom. She would avoid taking the kids to parks, beaches, barbecues—basically any location where the bathroom was not nearby. Her husband didn't hesitate or think twice about expressing his aggravation over the fact that he was inconvenienced by all this. Beverly was at a loss as to how she could deal with her present situation. She loved her husband, but had no idea how to address the downward spiral her relationship had taken. Obviously I could not share my entire book with her over the phone, but I did have a few suggestions.

First, I wondered if she had ever discussed the possibility of taking an antidepressant with her doctor. I thought that she may want to look into that because, as I knew from personal experience, chronic illness and the stress it can bring to a relationship can definitely lead to clinical depression. Second, I wondered if Beverly and her husband had ever considered seeing a counselor who was familiar with chronic illness and the resulting stress it added to one's relationship. Thirdly, I mentioned the need for and importance of clear, open, and honest communication in her relationship. These three options could go a long way in the process of helping the couple to recognize and address the relationship-destroying "Poor Me Attitude" that was being lived by both Beverly and her husband. Hopefully, this could help both her and her husband begin a discussion that would allow them to see the damage that was being done to their relationship as a result of a lack of compassion, misplaced anger, and poor communication between the two of them.

Now I would like to share my story with you because I wish to show you the stealth-like destructive ways in which this situation can destroy the strongest, most loving relationship. This true, firsthand account is my real-life story dealing with a marriage interrupted by multiple sclerosis. It could have been any chronic illness or disability and anybody's relationship, but my reason for writing this book is the same. My goal is to help others in a similar situation recognize and eliminate the growth of the relationship-destroying "Poor Me Attitude" that frequently accompanies chronic illness.

CHAPTER 1

My personal battle with multiple sclerosis:

In 1980, at the spry young age of eighteen, I was diagnosed with multiple sclerosis during my freshman year of college. I had been attending Johnson State College, located in Johnson, Vermont. Never in a million years would I have seen this one coming. I mean, I had just finished high school not more than a year earlier. During high school I played freshman baseball, in my junior year I played hockey, and during my senior year I was on the wrestling team. I was as healthy as the proverbial horse.

However, one Monday in March 1980, after what was then a pretty regular college weekend of partying, my body felt noticeably different. On this particular Monday, I mentioned to Steve, a friend in my dorm, that my hand had been completely numb all day. I first noticed the numbness in class that afternoon when I couldn't hold onto my pencil and later that evening I had the same problem trying to hold onto my eating utensils at the dining hall. Steve, or Witty, as he was known to his friends, thought that maybe I had a pinched nerve. The following day, I went to the local hospital in Mooresville. Following a full day of answering questions and numerous tests, the doctors could not find any reason for the numbness in my right hand. They sent me back to my dorm after telling me that the numbness was likely due to the stress of exams and the rigors of college life in general.

I remember thinking, that's a pretty lame diagnosis, but it was final exam season and I didn't have the time or strength to stress about this too. After a couple of weeks, the numbness seemed to increase rather than decrease, so I visited the larger teaching hospital in Burlington, where they were also unable to determine a cause for the numbness. At the time, I wasn't nervous or scared. I figured if the doctors couldn't find anything, it couldn't be that serious, right?

In May, I went home to Massachusetts for the summer break. During this time I visited a neurologist, Dr. Arthur Safran, who had an incredible bedside manner. You know how sometimes when you meet a doctor you can tell in the first few minutes that you're really going to like him or her? That was my experience with Dr. Safran. He was caring and compassionate. He explained himself extremely well, and went out of his way to make sure that I understood exactly what he was saying. The doctor performed a series of tests, including a CAT scan. The scan showed a number of plaques, or lesions, on my brain. These findings were consistent with a demyelinating condition, which would eventually help determine a diagnosis of multiple sclerosis. I say eventually because prior to the late 1980s a patient would only be diagnosed with MS when symptoms were experienced numerous times. For this reason, prior to the advent of the MRI scanner, which could clearly demonstrate damage to the myelin and central nervous system, a diagnosis of multiple sclerosis often took years. Myelin is the protective or insulating material surrounding nerve cells. Damage to the myelin can eventually result in the body's loss of neurological function.

Multiple sclerosis, "multiple" meaning many and "sclerosis" meaning scars or plaques, is a disease that has generally proven difficult to diagnose. When the plaques/scars are noticed in the brain or central nervous system for the first time, the diagnosis is usually one of a demyelinating condition. I was told that if the symptoms subsided or disappeared completely and returned at a later date, again and again, the condition was called multiple sclerosis.

So I left Dr. Safran's office that June day feeling pretty great, because I had just learned that I did not have multiple sclerosis, I had a demyelinating condition. At least that's what I took away from the discussion, because it would take time to see if the symptoms were going to come and go to make a positive determination of whether I had MS or not. Sadly, this eventually turned out to be my fate. I suffered numerous exacerbations of the disease and experienced a myriad of symptoms ranging from numbness, weakness, double vision, frequent loss of balance, and loss of portions of my visual field, just to name a few. Because no one, not a physician, family member or friend ever stepped up and said, the symptoms have come and gone several times, therefore you have MS, I just assumed that I did not have it. I suppose this was my own version of denial.

I'll never forget the day or where I was when I referred to my situation as a demyelinating condition in the presence of my father. I remember him stopping me and saying, "You have MS." I was so stunned to hear that. It should not have come as a shock to me, because I knew the symptoms had been coming and going for months. I knew that once an individual had been found to have a demyelinating condition and the symptoms came and went several times the condition was then labeled multiple sclerosis. That day I remember thinking, "Wow! I really have MS."

When something like that becomes reality it really hits you. I think I spent the rest of the day in my room, in tears, reading about multiple sclerosis in the *World Book* encyclopedia. In those days we didn't have the Internet, and the encyclopedia, if I remember correctly, just gave the worst-case scenario regarding the progression of the disease. As if it were yesterday, I can remember closing the encyclopedia and going to sleep that night believing that I was going to be in a wheelchair within a year, and that life was just going to go downhill from there.

During the second semester of my sophomore year of college the symptoms begin to flare up again. The numbness had become much greater in my right hand. So great, that I had to learn how to function proficiently using my left hand rather than my right. I spent much of the semester suffering from double vision. I walked around with one eye closed to eliminate seeing two of everything. I lived on campus with a bunch of great guys on the third floor of Governors South, who had a sense of humor much like my own. For a time every guy on the floor walked around with one eye closed or winking at one another. It really was a pretty humorous time in my life and it could have been miserable had it not been for the guys with whom I lived. I was blessed with the opportunity to have met and lived with each and every one of them.

That semester in 1981 was the last time I ever skied. Between my compromised vision and increased MS-related fatigue in my legs, I found myself skiing out of control more often than not. I could have continued to ski, but no longer at the same level as my friends or without jeopardizing the safety of others. Actually, I never skied close to the same high skill level as my buddies, Knoop, Squatch and Charlie all of whom were professional ski instructors for a decade or more. The strangest thing was that the more frequently that I skied the more inexperienced of a skier I appeared to be. This, like so many other things, became so frustrating. Remember, at this time I was not aware that I had MS and if I was, I had not yet admitted it to myself. Over the next year or so I acknowledged that I had multiple sclerosis, but because it was the relapsing remitting form (the symptoms came and went), I didn't believe my disability would progress. As I did in most cases throughout the next thirty-five years, when I lost the ability to perform one activity that interested me, I would find or develop another.

In college, I studied to become an ecologist or environmental scientist, working in the field, but because I had to avoid the heat of the outdoors, which exacerbated my symptoms, I pursued employment that would allow me to work indoors. In 1984 I began working as a quality assurance chemical technician for a company which produced powdered infant formula and other nutritional products. Not exactly ecology, but science is science. After about six years it became more difficult for me to be on my feet all day. My visual acuity had begun to further deteriorate, but most troublesome was my failing manual dexterity. I knew that I was eventually going to have to make a career move.

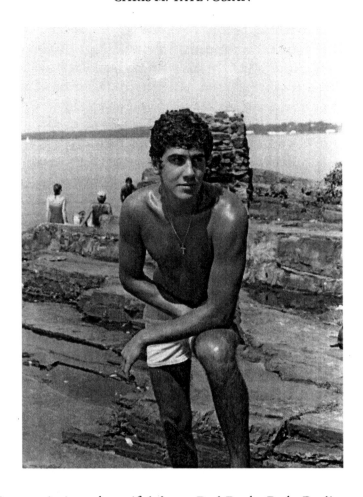

I was enjoying a beautiful day at Red Rocks Park, Burlington Vermont, during the summer of 1985.

In 1989 I went back to school and studied to be an adult educator. After all, if I was facilitating a class or speaking to a crowd no one would notice that I had MS, right? Many an audience probably assumed that I had a few too many drinks before class (just kidding). Jumping ahead a bit just to give you an example of how disease progression can be combated by tweaking or adjusting one's life, I'd like to share the following: During the early '90s I had a small business providing companies with occupational health and safety training in compliance with OSHA regulations. I remember standing in front of a group of about forty-five students, employees of a construction company. The group making up the class was a complete mix of employees from every department, blue-collar, white-collar, men and women alike. I was teaching with the aid of an overhead projector and I had my back to the screen for the most part, but as I spoke I occasionally looked at the overhead projection. A few moments into my presentation one of my students pointed out that the transparency was upside down. A simple sarcastic joke could easily cover up that blunder. In this game of MS you have to stay on your toes, smile. Can you imagine if I was easily embarrassed?

Luckily, I have a good sense of humor, which I have always used to keep busy, stay sharp, enjoy life, and entertain others. In college I had performed some stand-up back in the early '80s. I have always loved making others smile or, better yet, causing others to have a serious side-splitting belly laugh, a laugh that brings tears to their eyes; just ask the other chemists in the laboratory where I worked during the mid-1980s. Picture a laboratory filled with lab tables, testing equipment and instrumentation, fume hoods, emergency eye wash stations, and ten male and female technicians recently out of college for the most part. In setting the stage for the following scenario, I emphasize male and female technicians and emergency eyewash stations. These emergency eyewash stations, located at every sink in the lab, are stainless steel bowls with spigots to wash your eyes in the event something like a caustic chemical were to accidentally get in your eyes.

Add to this picture me standing at the sink, looking all professional in my white lab coat talking with Esther, one of the other chemists. We are standing with an eyewash station between us. I'm standing there working at the sink talking with Esther when I go to put my hand on the eye wash station, which just happens to be at the same height as Esther's chest. Can you guess where my numb hand ended up? That's right, like I was holding a grapefruit.

Everyone could tell by the appalled, almost frightened expression on my face that what I had just done was unintentional. I must have looked like I saw a ghost, because the entire lab, including Esther, burst out into a roar of laughter. I like to think that I was responsible for bringing a bit of comic relief, although unintentional at times, into what could have been a much too serious and stuffy work environment.

Bottom-line, we've got to learn to adjust to life and work with the gifts we've been given to best deal and cope with that which life so graciously serves up to us. If that gift is humor, maybe photography, crossword puzzles or sports, whatever it is, utilizing it to make the best life out of the life and time that you have been given is what it's all about. Plus, there's an incredibly beneficial physiological aspect associated with laughter. Doctors have shown that laughter increases the level of antibodies within the human body. This means by laughing, one increases his or her own body's ability to fight infection and disease, plus laughter is free and there is no trip to the pharmacy.

What is Multiple Sclerosis?

Here is my simplest explanation: MS is a disease of the central nervous systems (brain and spinal cord) whereby components of the immune system (T cells and white blood cells), which normally protect the body by attacking, destroying, and eradicating the body of foreign invaders like bacteria and viruses, go awry. For some unknown reason, the white blood cells do not recognize the myelin coating that surrounds the nerves' cells as one's own tissue. As a result, the white blood cells attack the myelin sheath. (The cause or trigger(s) continues to elude the medical community around the world.)

You could think of the nerve fiber as an electrical wire, and its myelin sheath as the protective plastic coating covering the wire. When the white blood cells attack the myelin sheath, they produce scars or plaques referred to as lesions, which interfere and inhibit nerve impulses from traveling to and from the brain. The severity and extent of the symptoms are determined by where in the central nervous system the damage to the myelin occurs.

The following is a list of the symptoms of multiple sclerosis that I have experienced over the years and the subsequent treatment(s) to relieve an exacerbation or attempt to slow disease progression. Over the past twenty-six years, since being diagnosed I have been on every pharmaceutical regiment. Starting years ago with prednisone and ACTH, I've undergone plasmapheresis, treatments with Solumedrol, Imuran, methotrexate, several months of Cytoxan, Betaseron, Avonex, Novantrone, and more. After 1988, I was in remission for three years following ten months of Cytoxan (chemotherapy), but nobody knows if that was the result of the drug treatment or just the natural course of the disease.

My Symptoms and Disease Management Timetable

Approx. Date	Symptom (s)	Treatment Method
1980	numbness of right hand	Prednisone
1981	numbness of right hand, numbness of right foot, double vision, blurred vision	ACTH
1983	numbness of right hand	Plasmapheresis
1988	numbness, blurred vision, reduced visual field, loss of balance, weakness	Chemotherapy and ACTH
1992	" " " "	Methylprednisolone
1993	numbness, reduced, blurred, shaking vision, weakness, loss of depth perception	Betaseron
1994	" " " "	Methylprednisolone
1995	now using a wheelchair at times, increased weakness, numbness, visual loss, tremor and cognitive losses	Methylprednisolone
1996	all symptoms continued to worsen slowly but steadily	Chemotherapy, Methylprednisolone
1997	" " " "	Avonex
1998	" " " "	Avonex
1999	" " " "	Avonex
2002	does not seem to help, substantial reversal of cognitive losses may be related to the Novantrone	Novantrone
2003	amazing improvements	Bee Venom Therapy (see Appendix)
2005	Since 2003, I have been stinging myself 20-40 times, three days, a week using live honeybees (see Appendix).	
2007	disease progression has resulted in continued neurological losses	Copaxone

If you have or know someone who has MS, you may want to read Appendix A, Bee Venom Therapy (BVT), which explores my miraculous experiences with this alternative therapy using Honeybees. Appendix B, on the other hand briefly explores and provides contact information for those desiring to know more about some of the more traditional, frequently prescribed and latest disease modification therapies.

CHAPTER 2
My Background

I grew up in Holliston, Massachusetts, on a cul-de-sac within an extremely safe suburban neighborhood—a neighborhood probably best described as your typical "Charlie Brown/Peanuts" type neighborhood filled with numerous fun-loving kids with no idea how dangerous the world could be. In the circle during the day we played baseball, street hockey, and built ramps for jumping with our bikes and at night we would play hide and go seek, capture the flag, and more. Many of us had mini-bikes, so we spent hours in the woods cutting trails and riding our dirt bikes by day, and at night during the summer, in those very same woods we would sleep out in our tree fort. We'd be up until the wee hours of the night talking about girls, telling scary stories and eating pounds of candy and other junk food purchased just for this event. What a simple and innocent time in my life. We were just a group of eight to twelve young kids, ranging from the age of about eleven to sixteen, enjoying the blessed and protected lives of innocence that our parents provided.

After high school, I attended Johnson State College in Johnson, Vermont. I chose Vermont because I loved the outdoors, enjoyed skiing and hunting, and most importantly, I wanted to study the environment. I could not have imagined a place more wild, beautiful and pristine as that of the Northeast Kingdom of Vermont. I had left behind suburban

Massachusetts, which was very nice, don't get me wrong, but it was like I had stepped into a postcard when I arrived in the Northeast Kingdom. Within a few short weeks I learned and experienced more about nature and the environment of the Northeast than I had in my previous eighteen years.

The campus of Johnson State College is nestled amongst the Green Mountains high above lush green meadows surrounded by the panoramic vistas and shadows of the numerous hills and snow-covered peaks. As the fall nights get colder the landscape, made up of pastoral valleys, forested hillsides, and mountain peaks, create an experience, an incredible visual experience no less, known as atmospheric inversion. I had heard about this phenomenon, but I had never seen it and had no idea of its grandeur. During the fall, in the morning, the heavy, dense cold air, mist, and clouds become trapped in the valleys beneath the warm, lighter air aloft. Until the morning sun heats up the air in the valleys, the clouds sit close to the ground creating an eerily beautiful picture for which words alone cannot do justice.

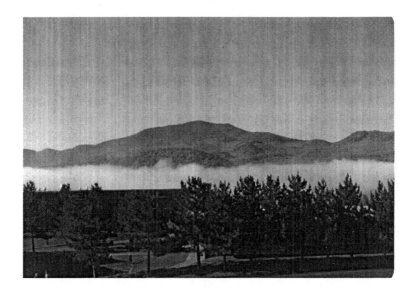

Many mornings in 1981, this was my view from my third-floor dorm room at Johnson state College, in the quiet town of Johnson Vermont. Notice the atmospheric inversion as the cooler air that came down off of Mount Mansfield during the night, warms and rises from the Valley of Johnson.

After graduation in 1983 with a B.S. in ecology and a minor in chemistry, I moved to Burlington, Vermont, with three buddies with whom I went to college. We remained roommates over the next seven years and would develop an awesome lifelong relationship. These three guys, "Kah-noop" (David Knoop), "Chah-lie" (Charles VanWinkle), and "Squatch" (David McCawley) were the best, and our friendship developed into a brotherhood that I will never forget. We were closer than most siblings, and we would have done and did do anything for one another.

Burlington, Vermont, is a great lakefront city, which I found difficult to leave. With four colleges and universities, approximately forty-five nightclubs, Lake Champlain for sailing, and plenty of mountains in the surrounding area for skiing, what twenty-year-old in his right mind could leave? Perhaps the more appropriate question would be: what twenty-year-old is in his right mind, anyway? Knoop, Charlie, Squatch (the boys), and I lived together in Burlington and the surrounding area for about seven years after living together on the same floor for four years in college. So we may have done a little partying together over the years; however, those memories aren't all that clear (smile).

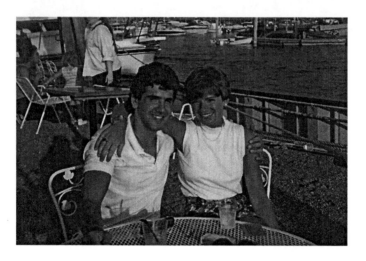

My friend, Hope and I were enjoying a summer afternoon back in 1987, at Breakwaters Restaurant on the waterfront in Burlington Vermont.

After moving to Burlington with "the boys" and completely enjoying a year off after college, in 1984 I found employment with a major nutritional and pharmaceutical giant, as a nutriceutical chemical technician. Don't get me wrong, I don't mean to imply that Knoop, Charlie, Squatch, and I found employment and stopped enjoying ourselves. On the contrary, now we showed less control because we could afford to go out two or three nights a week and splurge on some of the best toys.

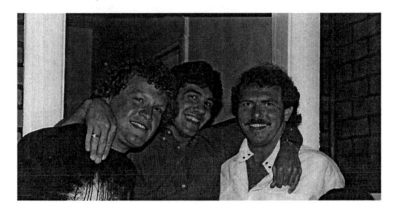

From left to right, a picture of me surrounded by my roommates Dave Knoop and Charlie Van Winkle, during a party at our 1987 home n Winooski Vermont.

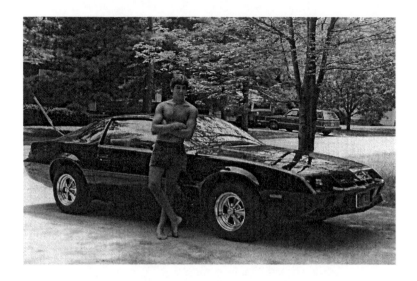

I am leaning against my Camaro during the summer of 1984, in the driveway of our (Dave, Charlie and my) home in South Burlington Vermont. If it seems like we moved a lot, we did. We actually moved six times in seven years for no particular reason, as far as you know.

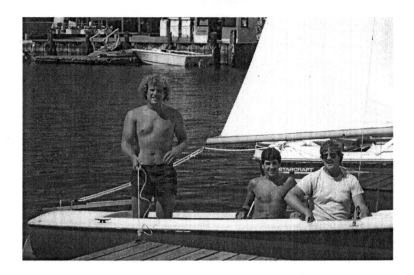

From left to right, about to disembark for the afternoon from Burlington Harbor in 1985, are Dave Knoop, me and Dave "Squatch" McCawley. Missing from the photo is our fourth roommate Charlie VanWinkle, behind the lens.

Between the four of us we had the best ski equipment, sailboards, a hot-looking new sports car, a motorcycle, and a sailboat. It wasn't "lifestyles of the rich and famous," but like that great comedian, Steve Martin, used to say, we enjoyed some "wild and crazy times."

I can remember sailing out of the beautiful Burlington Harbor with Knoop at the tiller and Charlie and me looking like prim and proper yachtsmen. I recall one of us jokingly asking, "I wonder what the poor people are doing today" with smiles on our faces. Then, after a full eight hours on the lake drinking beers in the hot summer sun, we sailed back into the harbor looking all sophisticated and hoity-toity—Not! As

I recall, the actual scenario went more like this: Knoop was now standing at the tiller trying to maneuver the boat into the harbor, in front of hundreds of weekend waterfront restaurant patrons and revelers who were eating and enjoying afternoon cocktails, when all of a sudden "Duke" (my nickname from college) and Charlie fell overboard inside the boat lane of the inner harbor. Of course, this took place right in front of the sign with the big red circle around the picture of a swimmer with a big red line through him.

Like the previous four years in college, the next seven years didn't look much different. Life resembled one long episode of Abbott and Costello interrupted by short bouts of seriousness. Laugh after laugh with great friends, my best friends, made what could have been a depressing and difficult decade the most joyous and memorable period of my single life,

Then in 1990, I received my "almost master's degree" from Trinity College, also in Burlington. I say it this way because the college never implemented the master's program in human resources dealing specifically with adult education prior to declaring bankruptcy and closing its doors. At that time, I began working as a subcontracted Occupational Safety and Health coordinator for a large corporation in Essex, Vermont.

I married Rachel, the woman of my dreams, in May 1992. Up until this time and into the first year of my marriage, I had been undergoing a remission of symptoms. This remission, which had been ongoing for more than five years beginning in 1988, coincided with a ten-month treatment protocol (once a month intravenous drip) of chemotherapy (Cytoxan). For the most part my MS was unnoticeable. I worked out in the gym four nights a week. I walked, drove my car, and clearly functioned normally and with few recognizable symptoms. I still had issues with my vision and fatigue, but to the outside world they were unnoticeable.

Rachel and I had begun dating in July 1990. We met through mutual friends at our health club where we both worked out. We went out on our first date on July 8, 1992. People were always impressed that I remembered the date of our first date—but don't be. July 8 just happened to be my birthday. It was a beautiful summer day, so we had lunch at the Queen City Tavern on the marketplace in Burlington, a marketplace designed and constructed by the same architect that designed Quincy Market in Boston. Therefore, the Burlington marketplace had much of the same nuance, character, and charm as that of Quincy Market in that they both had beautifully designed brick streets closed to vehicle traffic, decorative and historical statues, manmade fountains, outdoor cafes, and street vendors and artisans amongst the many beautiful shops and businesses. From there we went a couple of blocks down to the waterfront and sat out on the deck of the Burlington boathouse, overlooking Lake Champlain, where we enjoyed the view, a couple of cocktails, the warm sun, and a cooling breeze that was coming off the water. Our date continued throughout the entire day.

The city of Burlington had become my adopted home away from home since moving there in May 1983. It was so much like a resort town that you felt like you were at a resort on vacation miles away from reality. Later that afternoon, we went to the movies, where we saw Mel Gibson and Goldie Hawn in *Bird on a Wire*. Eventually, we dropped in on a good friend of mine, Steve Cusick. Steve was the main bartender at one of the hottest nightspots, the Chicken Bone Cafe, in downtown Burlington during the '80s and early '90s. So, I thought visiting Steve would be a good idea, plus it gave me the opportunity to show Rachel more of my personality. Stephen and I could play our sense of humor off of one another, and the mood was light, relaxed, and entertaining. It turned out to be a fantastic day. Rachel and I continued dating steadily for the next two years. For the longest time it seemed that we had so much in common that we couldn't get enough of one another, and we became inseparable. We did everything together. We attended all the annual events in Burlington, such as the midsummer Reggae Festival, the First Night New Year's Eve celebration, the Fourth of July celebration, the Burlington "ChewChew" festival (a three-day festival put on by the restaurants in the city), concerts taking place on the waterfront throughout the summer, watching road races, parades, and so much more. Together we also did so much with our son, Jesse (my stepson). Other than meeting and marrying Rachel, having the opportunity to be a father and participate in the process of raising Jesse was the best thing that ever happened to me.

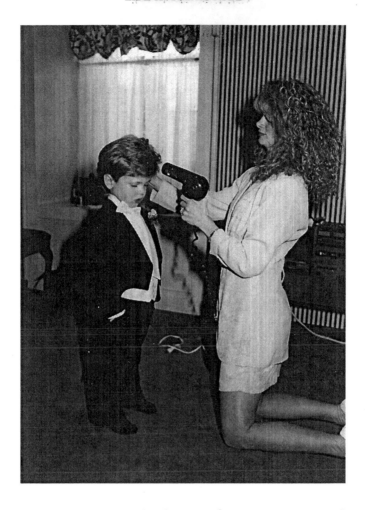

My stepson, Jesse Snyder, age five was getting ready to give his mother, Rachel, away in our April 1992 wedding.

Together, my wife and I took Jesse to see the Red Sox and Celtics play games down in Boston. We frequently attended Vermont Expos games (Burlington's junior league baseball team), visited Boston's science museum, aquarium, as well as many of the cities historical sites like Plymouth Plantation, Boston's Fanuel Hall, and so much more. Because I was such a big part of Jesse's development from the time he was three years old, Jessie developed my personality, mannerisms, and sense of humor. There's no greater reward than raising a child and seeing yourself when you watch and listen to him move through life.

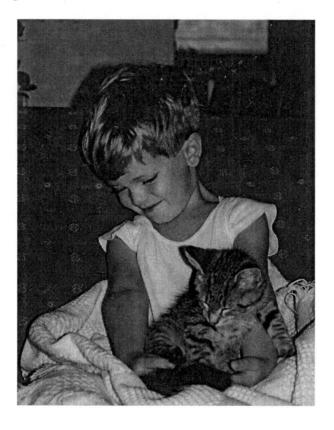

Jessie and Putty-Tat (evosian) preparing to start their day, June 1992.

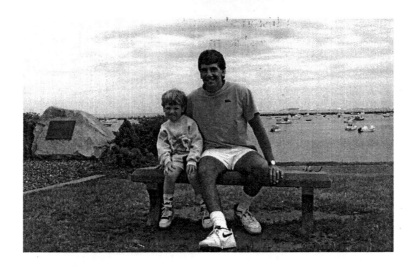

Jessie and I with Rachel behind the camera lens in Plymouth MA, 1993.

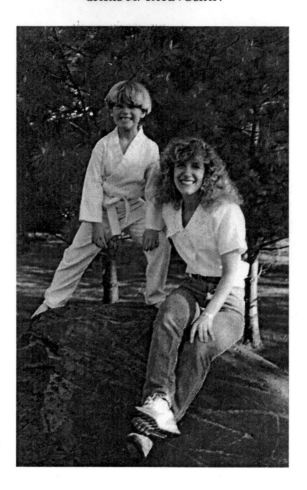

Jessie and Rachel in the backyard of our Essex Junction, Vermont condominium in 1994.

We enjoyed being a family and everything seemed to be going so well, but all good things must come to an end. I was laid off in 1993, and the resulting stress triggered a flare-up of my disease. The exacerbation was the worst that I had ever suffered.

I began to feel dizzy, extremely weak, and nauseous. I felt like I had the flu. Rather than subsiding, the symptoms worsened over the next two weeks. Eventually, I became so dizzy and unstable it was impossible for me to stand up. It was like the room was spinning. The fact that I did not have a fever and I felt like I was going to vomit but never did was not symptomatic of any flu that I had experienced previously. Finally, I felt like I had to go to the hospital. Because I could not move, and I was on the second floor of our condominium, I had to be removed from the house on a stretcher by emergency medical technicians and taken via ambulance to the hospital.

It turned out that I was actually undergoing an exacerbation of MS. This exacerbation, which caused damage to the brain stem, had to be treated intravenously with the steroid Solumedrol. As a result of this exacerbation, I became permanently disabled and unable to work. Of course, this added a whole new group of stresses to life, ranging from financial issues to the long battle for Social Security disability benefits. I discuss this in greater detail within Chapters Three and Four, which explore and deal with the damaging effects of worry and stress upon my relationship.

I returned home after a week-long stay in the hospital, and the exacerbation subsided to a certain extent. It would most likely take months before I would better understand what level of disability would be permanent. At the time I knew that I could not walk without a cane. I was legally blind. I could see, but it was like looking through a piece of Swiss cheese and parts of the picture were missing. My depth perception was severely compromised. Plus, now my eyes were shaking, so the view of my world would probably be best described as that of a tiny person in a snow globe.

Remember when you were a kid and you had one of those liquid and plastic snow-filled glass globes that you would turn upside down and shake to make the wintry scene come to life? That was the view of the world for me. The doctors explained that this condition was known as mystagmis, ironically as the result of my brain directing my eyes to move back and forth searching for the best view through that so-called "Swiss cheese."

Even though I was diagnosed with multiple sclerosis in 1980, the condition did not really affect my life dramatically until this exacerbation in May 1993. From that time, the disease just steadily progressed until 1995 when I had to stop driving because of vision problems and the inability to move my right leg quickly on and off the gas and brake pedals. At this point the disease was now being described by my doctors as "progressive" MS, whereas prior to this point the designation had been "relapsing remitting." The simplest explanation goes something like this: Progressive disease is just that. The disease worsens with little or no improvement, whereas the relapsing remitting form of the disease is one of flare-ups and partial to complete improvement.

One could allow MS to rule one's life; however, after letting the disease control my life for years, today I choose to look at MS and the cumbersome situations which it presents as a game. From the time I was a young child, I was deeply immersed in sports, sporting events, and competitive games. Not intending to brag or sound arrogant, I must say that I've won more games than I've lost. I intend to do the same thing with this so-called game of MS. Life is too short to worry about what may or may not happen. During my lifetime, I have had numerous friends that passed away in their twenties—some even younger—and they did not have a diagnosed illness. You just never know what's going to happen, especially in this day and age. All of us need to cherish every moment and thank God for the gift of each one.

In June 1993, I accepted Jesus Christ as my personal Lord and Savior, after having left the church after graduating from high school in 1979. After being away from the church for more than ten years, I was invited out to church by my friend and co-worker, Chuck DiShino. Chuck knew I was suffering from MS and that it had recently progressed.

For several weeks Chuck continued to tell me about and invite me to visit the Christian church to which he belonged. I was brought up Catholic, and it seemed like a lifetime since I had last attended a church of any kind. I finally gave in and grudgingly got out of bed for church. I say it this way because it's not difficult to come up with an excuse for staying in bed when it comes to going to church. At least that's the way I felt back then.

My first Sunday back, on the floor of a small, cold church in the old north end of Burlington, Vermont, I fell to my knees and gave my life to Jesus Christ. There have been times that I have fallen away from the church, but I can honestly say that since moving back to Massachusetts in 2002 I have found the most incredible home at the First Congregational Church of Hopkinton, and Sunday morning can not come quick enough. The rededication of my life to God has provided me with the most incredible levels of strength, perseverance, character, and hope.

Personal notes, thoughts and memories, concepts and Ideas, that I would like to put into practice:

In the lives of any one of us change is inevitable, but change ambushes the lives of the disabled, those suffering from chronic illness as well as the lives of their loved ones who many times serve as the caregivers. The problem is that the illness and living with the hardship brought on by the illness often brings to light a particularly negative exchange. In many young relationships this may be the first time such a mean-hearted display has shown itself in the relationship. As you grow and change, you have to be aware of how your change affects the lives of those you love. You can become oblivious to the needs of everyone around you as a result of falling into the depressing, hurtful downward spiral of the "Poor Me Attitude." No one knows this better than me. I just wish I had someone to slap me upside the head and yell, "Snap out of it! It's not all about you!!!"

As an individual suffering from multiple sclerosis, I want to help you avoid making the relationship-destroying mistakes that I made. By recognizing how your attitude, actions, stress, and depression affects your physical, mental, and verbal interactions with the person who is your closest loved one and best friend, you will have the knowledge and awareness to recognize and stop the development and cancerous growth of the "Poor Me Attitude" actions. After reading this book, I hope you will become better equipped to deal with your situation more positively. I intend to help you identify the "Poor Me Attitude," and through awareness avoid the stealth-like relationship-destroying characteristics of that "Poor Me Attitude." Through awareness you can have a proactive rather than a reactive approach to many of the difficult situations you may face. Because the proactive approach is generally positive and the reactive approach is more likely to illicit negativity, resulting in frustration and anger, the proactive or positive approach is obviously much more beneficial in the process of growing a healthy relationship.

Why is it that it is easier to forgive a stranger than your spouse? I mean, out of frustration we often find—at least I did—that it is so much easier to hurt our spouses, family members or partners. Unlike your spouse or partner, you aren't nearly as emotionally invested in a stranger. I know that when I verbally attacked my wife or she me, it really hurt. Part of the hurt comes from knowing that your spouse is well aware of exactly what will hurt you and uses that knowledge with the intention of causing pain and distress. The closeness that we develop with our partner provides easy access to a cachet of intimate knowledge into the innermost thoughts, feelings, and emotions of our spouse/partner. For the sake of your relationship, this information should stay private and not be used as hurtful weapons against one another. If this does happen consciously, this painful behavior must not be allowed to continue, or worse, simply allowed to be forgotten like it never happened. When we do end up fighting with one another and intentionally hurting each other we must have the strength to address the situation, apologize, and forgive one another. The situation cannot be fully resolved until you both have agreed as to how the situation would best be handled in the future in order to avoid this and similar hurtful behaviors from happening again.

If we look to the word of God, we learn that the apostle Peter denied and disappointed Jesus and we learn from Jesus when we ask ourselves, how did our Lord react to disappointment? When our Savior was being judged, persecuted, and facing death, Peter denied knowing Him before the Roman soldiers. Scripture says, "And the Lord turned and looked at Peter...so

Peter went out of the garden and wept bitterly," Luke 22: 61-62. Think about this. The Lord turned and looked at Peter. What did Peter see when his eyes met that of his persecuted and soon to be executed savior? Was it disappointment or anger? As justified as that would have been, when Peter's eyes made contact with those of the Lord, in that brief moment he saw the undying and boundless love and forgiveness of Christ. That's right. Peter saw nothing but love and forgiveness in that glance. Remember this the next time you and your spouse or partner disagree; remember the Lord's reaction is the perfect reaction, one which you must strive to emulate. Stun your spouse with love.

Know what to look for and how to recognize and identify the obvious and destructive "Poor Me Attitude " actions, which can often be downright mean, selfish, degrading, and controlling. The earlier that you are able to recognize these actions, the sooner you can work on repairing and rebuilding your relationship; otherwise, the relationship could likely be destined for miserable, hate-filled failure.

You must reduce, if you cannot eliminate completely, the cumulative effects of your depression, anger, and frustration. This will not be an easy task, but there are many resources and options available to assist you with this process. There is counseling to which I have devoted an entire chapter (see Chapter Seven), pharmaceutical drugs, doctors both mental and physical, and remember, talking openly and frequently with your partner regarding your problems, fears, and concerns is vital for the success of any relationship.

The first thing to recognize—and I know this because I missed it when it would have made a difference—is that seeing a counselor who deals with chronic illness, seeing any physician and taking a plethora of prescription drugs including antidepressants, though extremely beneficial for the individual suffering from the ailment, provides no relief for one's spouse or partner. The antidepressant Zoloft was a godsend for me. It never occurred to me how helpful it could have been for my spouse. When I think about it, it should not have been my responsibility anyway. You would think that a physician may have made that suggestion. After all, I have seen a few in my day.

Counseling, prescription drugs, it was all for me, when it should have been for *us*. In hindsight, which again is, of course, twenty-twenty, the concept of treating "us" rather than me alone is probably the most significant step in healing and protecting your relationship. Don't lose sight of this point. After all, in a healthy relationship any other problems are best treated as problems that must be addressed by the couple or the "us."

It's too late and very sad, but I recognize my biggest mistake and the needs and concerns of my ex-wife more after the divorce than I did while we were married. Why is that? Not because I know and understand her wants and needs that much better today and not because I hope to redeem myself. No, it's because I want you to recognize and avoid making the same relationship-destroying mistakes. Looking back, it's easy to recognize that my biggest problem was that I acted like my problems outweighed the importance of any problem or concern my ex-wife had. If this part of my life had been made into a movie that could be rewound and viewed on the big screen, my actions would be painfully embarrassing to watch. Looking back, not only is it hard to believe, but it's embarrassing to think that I was acting this way and never realized it. I did not see the immature prima donna that was me, who felt the world owed him everything.

CHAPTER 3
The "Poor Me Attitude"

What is this "Poor Me Attitude"? Without intervention and change, the loss of one's self-worth leads to an increase in anxiety, depression, anger, and loneliness, which ultimately will lead to the destruction of your relationship if those feelings are left to grow. The "Poor Me Attitude," as I refer to it, is really nothing more than a controlling attitude that started out with me unconsciously using my weakness, loneliness, and feelings of inadequacy to get what I needed. Because I felt so weak, alone, and inadequate, I would frequently lash out over trivial things.

For example, I expended a lot of energy cleaning up after myself during the day and because it was so taxing for me to do this, I would become very upset with my wife when she did something as minor as leaving her coffee cup on the counter in the morning rather than putting it in the dishwasher. After a while, the frustration of struggling both mentally and physically turned into anger and nastiness. I don't know when it started, but somewhere along the line I began to treat anger as a weapon. To manipulate my wife I attacked with sharp words, knowing that this behavior frequently resulted with my wife completing some task around the house that I foolishly thought needed immediate attention. Such a reaction did not display power; rather, it displayed my weakness.

A disability can result in such a dramatic change in one's personality and disposition that it more often than not is the cause of a couple's breakup or divorce. Not long ago, I learned from a friend that her mother and father's divorce was the result of that exact situation. Her father had become disabled after having suffered a stroke. He became so bitter, nasty, and filled with misdirected anger toward his wife that both his and her lives became filled with nothing but misery. They eventually divorced.

When I was struggling, my mood was one of nastiness. All my actions had become hidden agendas. My anger and nastiness developed into a learned technique for achieving my hidden agenda. At one point during my marriage I recall my wife saying that she tried to do everything to please me in an attempt to avoid upsetting me. Of course, she told me this so that I would be sympathetic and understanding. As a result, I thought I was being more understanding, but I had also learned that expressing anger was a way of getting what I wanted from her. I was guilty of angrily expressing frustration and hardship likely resulting from the embarrassment of my physical losses such as strength, energy, and simple motor skills. Furthering this problem were the larger culprits: my mental and emotional losses, the loss of my self-esteem, and the development of cognitive difficulties. This behavior became the norm. In my mind I didn't recognize my relationship-damaging and selfish behavior because my personal struggle to function was all-consuming of both my mental and physical strength. I mean, come on, every simple daily task like tying my sneaker, standing up in the shower or holding an eating utensil became an embarrassing struggle.

Whether we want to admit it or not, the damage to our own egos can cause so much anger. Unfortunately, much of it is misplaced anger, and who is the unfortunate recipient of that anger? That's right, I'll take "my wife" for $500, Alex. If someone, somehow, had been able to help me recognize I was acting that way so that I could have changed my behavior and stepped out of that "it's all about me" fog, my marriage might still be intact today. Having a chronic illness or disability is horrible, tragic, and unfair. If you surround yourself in that fog of misery and self-pity, you may just be involved in a tragic accident, the result of which will be the tragic loss of your relationship, marriage or family.

Every relationship has its ups and downs. There will be arguments, disagreements, and fights. Tempers will flare, thoughtless comments may fly, and the wrong tone of voice or even a look meant to hurt causes a wound. Inevitably, the accumulation of wounds will likely cause the death of the relationship. Are you ready to lose the love of your life? My hope is that by reading about my experiences you will be able to recognize and halt your own relationship-destroying behaviors.

Here are a few examples from my past, which I hope will better illustrate this relationship-destroying mechanism.

Had I been aware of this controlling "Poor Me Attitude" and unselfishly changed my ways, my marriage could be alive and well today. I frequently started projects that needed to be done around the house, knowing that it would be impossible for me to complete the task. I was attempting to help out around the house, but if you're familiar with MS, you know that once you start any project it doesn't take long for the monster known as MS-related fatigue to rear its ugly head. The monster literally renders one useless. It may become impossible to move or maybe you lose your vision or ability to carry out a thought process. Whatever it is, it's scary, unnerving, even embarrassing.

By starting this or any project, it was my intention to be helpful and at the same time boost my extremely low level of self-worth. As you will learn in the following examples, the outcomes were anything but helpful and pleasing.

In September 1998, at the height of the relatively new dot com frenzy, my wife began looking for work in the Boston area. At that time I had not realized it, but my marriage had been strained for sometime. My family lived in the suburbs of Boston and Rachel felt that if she could find work in the Boston area, being closer to my family could alleviate some of the burden caring for me placed on her. I thought her idea was great for a couple of reasons. First, just the idea of living in close proximity to my parents, grandparents, aunts and uncles, my two sisters and their husbands was mentally uplifting as I had positive relationships with my family and extended family. In turn, living in close proximity tapped into a potentially incredible support system, thus possibly alleviating some of Rachel's care-giving responsibilities. My disease had obviously progressed to the point where the role of caregiver was too much for one person, especially if that individual was working ten and eleven hours a day, as my wife had been doing for several years.

One drawback causing us to rethink the idea of moving to Massachusetts was the reality of moving Jesse away from both his father and his friends just when he was beginning high school. We thought starting high school was difficult enough, and moving Jesse to a new school in a new state really intimidated him. Rachel and I felt that he might be harassed and teased by the high school students in the city schools of Boston, Massachusetts, and this would be a difficult transition after being raised and schooled in a sheltered Vermont community.

After mulling over our options, we decided to put our house on the market, to see what might happen; if our house sold, we would then decide if moving near Boston was our next step. Within weeks —I believe it was January, 2000 —a young couple offered to purchase our home. One Sunday morning as Rachel was looking through the newspaper, she found a listing with a scheduled open house that afternoon. Though the property seemed to be out of our price range, we thought we'd take a ride to see it, and get out of the house for a little while that afternoon. My wife occasionally had mentioned that she imagined herself at this stage of life to be living in a more spacious, upscale dwelling rather than our starter home. I felt the same way, so off we went. The listed house was located in Essex Junction, an approximate three minute drive from where we had lived for the past decade. The neighborhood was a new development and we had never driven there before. When we turned off the main road into this new development, we both started laughing: what we saw was too good to be true. Keep in mind, this house was located less than a mile from our home and yet we had never bothered to drive this particular street because it was a dead end. What we found —the house and neighborhood —was beyond our imagination.

My wife and I turned and looked at one another; simultaneously we exclaimed, "Pleasantville!" If you have seen the movie *Pleasantville,* which was released in the mid-1990s, I am sure you now have a mental picture of the neighborhood. For those reading this book who have not seen the movie, I'll briefly give a description.

In the movie, all the neighbors were friendly and helpful, almost to the point of being sickening. People were walking the street, sharing friendly hellos and friendly greetings. The kids were outside playing or selling lemonade on the roadsides, while the adults helped one another with projects around their homes. Others were having conversations in the road, in the middle of the cul-de-sac, or across their yards. Still others were complementing others on their beautiful gardens or lawns, or how incredible little Johnny was playing in Little League, or that they had read in the local paper that little Susie made the honor role, again. A fabulous time warp, visually linked to *Pleasantville* and a simpler more caring time reminiscent of an era long past, had taken place when we turned onto the road.

On the right side of the road were well manicured lawns abutting beautiful single-family homes. On the left, was a playground with swings, a jungle gym and a slide. Near the playground, was an area of picnic tables and barbecue grills if the neighbors wanted to get together and socialize. Beyond the picnic area were two tennis courts and a Little League baseball field. At this point along the right side of the road, there was a cul-de-sac surrounded by five beautiful homes, one of which had a big sign on the front lawn advertising an open house. As we drove closer to the house, we could see that the backyard sloped down and two large wraparound decks were attached to the back of the house. From the decks of this magnificent home, Rachel and I could see a big red barn adjacent to a beautiful pond farther down the road. Later on we would learn that the pond was stalked with fish, the barn was home to a mother fox and her four pups, and deer journeyed out of the woods into the backyards. Like a picturesque postcard, this vista would eventually be the view from our back decks.

Rachel and I purchased this wonderful white three-bedroom home and moved in on May 5, 2000. We loved it. The master bedroom suite with a large walk-in closet was on the first floor; the first floor was roomy, with a wide-open floor plan. A second bathroom, kitchen, dining and living room completed the spacious first floor which opened up onto the decks. This first floor plan was perfect for me. Everything was accessible with the use of my walker. Two large bedrooms and another full bathroom made up the second floor. The purchase was a new start to a life which had been growing more and more difficult both mentally and physically.

Unfortunately, yet perhaps predictably, the excitement of moving into our dream home in Pleasantville was only a temporary fix to what was, and would become again, a stressed and troubled marriage. For several months after moving into our dream house, we lost track of the real reason we had looked into moving to Boston in the first place. Remember, the move was planned as an attempt to alleviate the hardships and workload falling on my wife's shoulders. It was not long before I started beginning projects and utilizing hidden agendas just as I had in our last home.

For example, our new purchase, this beautiful three year-old house that was in fantastic condition, really needed nothing. Because it had been lived in for three years, our new house only needed minor cosmetic and aesthetic improvements. One afternoon I took it upon myself to begin shampooing the carpets and another when I started staining the deck. The deck was faded. Perhaps it hadn't been stained for three years and the carpets just needed to be washed. Not because the rugs looked dirty, it was just to give us peace of mind so that we could play a game on the floor, lay around watching television or play with the dog without being concerned with what had previously been spilled on the carpet by the previous owners.

On both occasions I was unable to finish the project because of MS-related fatigue. When my wife arrived home from work, she had to complete the projects. The first few times that my wife arrived home from work only to find me collapsed on the floor, she would have to immediately take over where I left off. I say immediately, because I was a bear. I suppose that I learned that I could get my wife to complete any project around the house or yard with this same scenario of using started projects as hidden agendas with the intention of having my wife complete the project. I did not set out with this as my intended plan. I'm sorry for having put my ex-wife through this, and I'm embarrassed and ashamed. I don't know if this process was something that only I have experienced. I have to think that it was not. Acting this way was not my original intention and in any case it's important to be aware of the possibility that you may be guilty of doing the same thing.

Have you ever been awakened by the occasional slamming of a broken screen door or shutter being slammed against the house by the wind? Just when you start to fall into a deep sleep again, slam! the torment continues. In a relationship there will be times when your husband, wife or child will get on your nerves. That's inevitable. Maybe your spouse wants you to do something like cut the grass, stain the deck or shampoo the rugs. It is usually some inconsequential task that has seemingly become an irritant that requires immediate attention. Slam, slam, slam!

In my case, I'm sure that my wife felt that the easiest way to eliminate the slamming irritant was to appease me by addressing the situation about which I was complaining or upset. In every relationship there will be times when one person will drive the other a little nuts, but that's just part of life. It is when you go overboard and constantly cause stress, anxiety, and misery that you create a tension that will destroy even the closest relationship. When you have a disagreement it's important and essential that you have the grace to give in with a smile and think about what is really important.

There are so many ways that the controlling "Poor Me Attitude" sneakily moves into your life and relationships. I say sneakily because I didn't realize how controlling I was being and how I was selfishly making life all about me. Here are a few experiences from my life that will make the controlling nature of the "Poor Me Attitude" actions easier to recognize.

I recall shortly after moving into our new home, my wife was invited over to the next-door neighbors for a Tupperware party, and I became upset and made her feel guilty for wanting to go and leave me home alone. We owned several cabinets full of Tupperware containers, and I had been alone all day while my wife was at work, so when she got home it was my first opportunity to interact and spend time with another adult. What I didn't recognize was going to a Tupperware party at the neighbors was not about purchasing more Tupperware containers, it was an opportunity for my wife to socialize with the new neighbors. Unlike me, you have to recognize that your partner has needs. Whether you intentionally or unintentionally are being controlling, this behavior—which could be legitimately construed as selfish—can be extremely damaging to your relationship. Some of you reading this may be saying, just a minute, your wife was also being selfish. Today I would say that it's a two-way street and you both have to reach a compromise with an outcome that provides for mutual happiness.

I often failed to recognize my wife's need for time to herself, because my growing self-pity and my lack of self-worth blinded me to everyone else's needs. For instance, on Thursdays my wife would receive her *People* magazine in the mail. When she got home from work, she would immediately sit down and begin reading it. Of course, that was upsetting to me because I wanted to interact with her after being alone all day. I did not recognize how selfish and controlling I was being. In my mind my loneliness made it "all about me." Many people returning home from work need ten or twenty minutes alone to wind down from their workday. My ex-wife was doing just that, and I selfishly made it all about me.

Lastly, my need to get out of the house became an issue. Looking back, I recognize that I never got over the issue of losing my independence and that loss created a lot of anger. At the time I didn't know it, but I was placing the burden of getting me out of the house, whether it was to go shopping or just sightseeing, on my wife. Many times she would have just returned from grocery shopping or running an errand, and I would be waiting alone at home, and as soon as she walked in the door, I would ask her if she wanted to go out and do something. Of course, at that time the last thing she wanted to do was go out again. I would become upset and angrily let her know that "poor me" needed to get out of the house and do something, anything.

I should not have made getting me out of the house her responsibility. You and I both know that there were many ways that I could have gotten out to do things. There were many options, less convenient, but still many options existed. I could have gotten rides from friends or called the local bus service for the disabled. The bottom line was that I really wanted to get out with my wife. As I said before, had I been aware of the "Poor Me Attitude" actions and unselfishly changed my ways, my relationship could be alive and well today.

Of course, I mustn't forget the "Shirley factor." Shirley

was our sweet, loving, and, when left alone, destructively over-anxious dog. So the dog played a major role in my inability to leave the house. Shirley, if I had to take an educated guess, was a bloodhound and whippet mix that went to work with my wife two days during the week, and she stayed home with me the remaining three. Rachel was employed by a progressive, employee-friendly snowboard manufacturer, which allowed its employees to bring their dogs to work. One could walk into the plant any day of the week and find twenty to thirty dogs sitting at their masters' cubicles or wandering the halls. The animals were a pleasure and he provided for a comfortable relaxed work environment. There was little or no barking and very few accidents. These were well-trained dogs that had been brought up with one another and coexisted extremely well or they were not allowed back on the premises. It was amazing to watch, and the occasional cat tossed into the mix didn't even cause a stir.

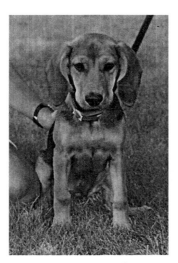

Shirley 1994

Our dog, Shirley, suffered from separation anxiety and when left alone would rip through the house like a destructive cyclone. During the first year, I did everything I could to give up the dog, but my wife couldn't part with her. One evening, back in 1994 when Shirley was still a puppy, my wife and I went out, leaving the dog home alone. When we returned home just four hours later, the dog had ripped the shades off the windows, severely scratched the door, ripped moldings from the wall, and attempted to eat through the sheet-rocked walls. If our condominium had not been constructed of brick, she probably would have gotten out.

We tried everything to correct the dog of this problem with little or no success. As a result, three days a week I was pretty much tied to the house. At one point, I said to my wife, "Either the dog goes or I go." My wife's response was, "But I love that dog." Jokingly I said, "Where does that leave me?" We just laughed.

Occasionally I would leave the dog with the neighbors and occasionally we even got a dog sitter. That's right, I said a dog sitter. When I was alone with the dog, I loved her company, but I frequently had to turn down going out with friends during the afternoon because I couldn't leave the dog alone. The dog was such a comfort and so damn cute, but because she could not be left alone I was tied to the house. Over time I could tell that I was becoming more depressed. I started sleeping the mornings away. I was easily frustrated, aggravated, and quick to anger. For the most part, I was not a pleasure to be around. It was like I had aged thirty years and become a grumpy old man. I realized how depressed I was becoming and how the depression was affecting my marriage, but I felt trapped as if there was nothing I could do?

If I knew when I was married what I know now, I would still be married to the woman of my dreams. Even several years after my divorce, it saddens me to think about what was lost. My ex-wife, Rachel, was an incredible wife and mother. She was extremely intelligent, driven, commonsensical, and like me, so funny at times. For the longest time we had the greatest relationship, but living with me and my physical and mental changes just became too much. It's too late for me, but it's not too late for you to save your marriage or relationship. It's a cliché, but it's true, "you don't know what you've got 'til it's gone." So let's work together to prevent the loss.

CHAPTER 4
Clear and Open Communication

If the writing of this book helps just one couple save their relationship, it will have been time well spent. I want to help you see what it is that you are doing to your relationship, spouse, family or partner by acting like you are the only one suffering as a result of your illness, injury, and/or disability. Remember, it's also extremely painful for the healthy partner to see his or her loved one struggling, having difficulty or in pain. "It's Not All About You" and the repetitiveness of your "Poor Me Attitude" and the replaying of your physical difficulties is not only a depressing drain on you, but also on the loved ones experiencing life with you on a daily basis.

During the course of a chronic illness like multiple sclerosis, as well as many others such as the long-term struggles of a disability of paralysis, the effects of a stroke, blindness, and the like, your spouse/partner comes to understand what you are experiencing and feeling. You don't need to describe it to them on a daily basis, but if you feel that you do need to do this, communicate and share with your partner why it is that you feel the necessity to do so. Remember, I was looking for my wife's opinion on whether she thought I was having an exacerbation and in need of an appointment with my neurologist. The problem developed and grew because of the lack of clear communication on my part. Looking back, I'm sure my ex-wife thought I was just complaining, and at the very least the process became tiresome, exacerbating the misery for the both of us. I can't stress enough the importance of clear and open communication. Clear, compassionate communication can prevent so many disagreements that can lead to major arguments that are altogether avoidable. Reduce your stress with communication.

"It's Not All About You." Remember to recognize all the good things the healthy spouse/partner has done and continues to do in order to make life easier for you. When it came to keeping our family and home running smoothly, my ex-wife was amazing. There was never an item that you needed that couldn't be found in the house. Whether it was a Band-Aid, battery, particular salad dressing or insect repellent it could be located with ease. I never knew anyone who could keep such a well-prepared home. I frequently told others what an excellent job she did providing for my stepson and me.

My wife was everything I ever wanted, she was everything I ever needed, she was everything to me, and I let that slip away by forgetting about her needs and making it all about me. It was so infrequent that I let her know how incredible I thought she was, and how thankful I was for her efforts to make my life as easy as possible. Of course, when I was struggling, which was frequently, I always complained about what could be done to make life easier for me. The complaints could have been about things like how difficult it was for me to get something out of the refrigerator or cabinet because of how things were put away. Because of my hardship and misery I did not hesitate to express angrily what I thought could have or should have been done to make my life easier.

I know probably better than most that when you're struggling it's difficult to calmly and politely share a suggestion designed to make your lives easier in the future. It's not likely that you're going to be handing out compliments of any kind in the middle of your misery and frustration, but it's important to make a note between the two of you to come back and address this situation when cooler heads prevail. This means that you are first going to have to agree and come to grips with the fact that things will get heated at times within every relationship. Therefore, a system of rational communication leading toward a mutually satisfying resolution of the situation must be developed. This system should allow the involved parties to come back and revisit the situation using a calm and structured approach, with the primary goal being a resolution that will prevent this and other similarly destructive situations from occurring in the future.

I would suggest both parties make a written note to themselves, so that when you encounter this situation, you and your partner can calmly discuss how to reduce or eliminate your struggles and miscommunications. If you have difficulty writing, I recommend purchasing a small handheld tape recorder. This device will enable you to quickly and conveniently record and later recall your thoughts for discussion with your partner. In most cases, a simple solution will accommodate the problem; however, other situations will arise that can best be addressed with the assistance of a counselor. For example, as a result of my difficulty walking I would frequently trip on doormats and small area rugs, causing me to become quite upset. At this point, I was of course actually mad at the MS, but you cannot take your frustration out on the MS, so your loved one(s) becomes the recipient(s) of your anger and nastiness.

After nine years of doing this, unsurprisingly I'm no longer married. Please be aware of this action and together seek the help of a counselor. Awareness of, and providing attention to, your relationship-destroying actions are the keys to saving your relationship. It's funny, but the song "Little Moments" performed by country music star Brad Paisley eerily displays precisely many hurtful situations and missed opportunities to show my wife what she really meant to me. Here, allow me to demonstrate what I mean by using the song's lyrics to make things clearer.

Following the paraphrased song lyrics, in parentheses you will see my real-life experiences. My goal here is to share with you my real-life interactions with my then wife so that you can see how foolishly I reacted to the eerily similar situations presented in the song lyrics. I realize that this is just a song designed to tug at one's heartstrings in order to sell albums, a marketing technique and a successful one at that. However, I want you to become aware of the selfish mistakes that I blindly made so that you can catch yourself before you do the same.

First, Brad Paisley sings about how he reacted to his wife backing his truck into something. He responds by letting us know that he couldn't even remember what it was she backed into and said he couldn't even act like he was mad, because she looked so damn cute. He sings: "I live for little moments like that."

My wife got into a small fender bender and my first response to her was not, "Are you all right?" It was: "How much damage is there to the car?" I must have been struggling miserably to have reacted in this manner. I know this happened, but looking back it doesn't make sense or seem possible to have reacted so inconsiderately with such callousness. I was obviously in a different state of mind, because today I cannot imagine having acted so selfishly with little or no regard for the feelings and safety of my then wife.

Personal notes, thoughts and memories, concepts and Ideas, that I would like to put into practice:

Second, Paisley sings about how last year on his birthday his sweetheart lost all track of time and burnt the cake. He took her in his arms and tried not to let her see him laugh. He sings, "I live for little moments like that."

One day my wife spent all afternoon making me a special dessert, and she ruined it by overcooking it. I reacted by getting upset with her. Again, where was my sense of reality and appreciation for what was important in life?

Third, he sings about how his sweetheart misread the directions and they were driving around holding hands while they were lost. Again, he says, "I live for little moments like that."

I was found to be legally blind in 1995. After that time, my wife always drove, and like anyone can, she occasionally got lost, missed an exit, or made a wrong turn. I would become extremely frustrated with her, making her feel bad. I understand that it's only a song and perhaps Mr. Paisley reacts a bit differently in real life, but I was easily angered and frustrated nine out of ten times. I know that I was so easily angered because I was struggling and suffering. Look where it got me. I pray that by sharing my real life experiences and unacceptable reactions with you, that you will be able to become more aware of your own unacceptable behaviors and work to eliminate or at the very least change them.

You may be physically and or mentally weak, but you must still express love, show your gratitude, praise, and make life pleasurable, not more miserable, for your spouse. We all know that this can be extremely difficult for even the healthiest relationships. All too often it proves to be impossible for all too many couples. So in a marriage that has been interrupted, so to speak, by chronic illness or disability, requiring one spouse/partner to be the caregiver for the other, requires thoughtful adjustments. From experience, I can tell you that the individual suffering the chronic illness or disability is likely to feel anger and depression, which consciously or unconsciously develops into what I call the "Poor Me Attitude." Both partners must consciously be unselfish, be understanding, provide one another with special attention, be respectful of one another, and most importantly, communicate clearly and openly.

Let me give you an example of what I mean because communicating clearly and openly sounds obvious, right? Yes but no, because when you're not in a rational state of mind, the obvious is no longer obvious. Everyone deals with conflict, and a healthy dose of conflict is fine. When I was married and struggling, just about every word out of my mouth was adversarial, which sparked conflict. I'm so much more aware and in control of it today, but if I'm not careful, on occasion I'll slip back into my old ways.

Nothing better demonstrates how difficult it is to stay calm, think rationally, and remain caring and loving toward those who mean the most to you when the ever-changing stresses of living with a chronic illness or disability are taking their toll on your own frame of mind better than what happened to me yesterday. I am living at home with my parents six years after my divorce, writing a book which is clearly about recognizing the problems and conditions that can lead to the destruction of a relationship resulting from the added stresses placed on that relationship as a result of one of the partners having a chronic illness or disability. Having lost my marriage, obviously I am an expert in this area right? Not!

Different caregiver, same problem continues:

Occasionally my relationship with my mother, who for the most part has taken on the role of caregiver, becomes very tumultuous and reminds me of how easily I became upset and in a way verbally abusive toward my wife when I was married.

Although I am aware of the "poor me" behavior that played a major role in the destruction of my marriage, I occasionally find myself falling back into the trap of acting similarly. Yesterday for example, It was a very warm and humid evening and I had been upstairs working on the computer in my air-conditioned office all day when I decided to go downstairs around seven o'clock for dinner. As I began to go downstairs, I was hit by a wall of heat and humidity in the part of the house that was not air-conditioned. Heat (as little as an increase of one-thirty-second of one degree) and humidity can actually shut down the functioning of the neurological system in ninety percent of the people suffering with MS. I fall into that category of sufferers. By the time I had worked myself down the steamy stairwell, I was a mess. On the first floor of the house the air conditioner was running, but the sliding glass door was open and the slight increase in warmth and humidity after spending a few minutes in the steamy stairwell was enough to ruin my evening as well as my mother's and those about to join us for dinner.

By the time I had entered the kitchen, my vision was almost gone, my hands felt like baseball gloves, and I couldn't support my torso or maintain my balance. I immediately lashed out because the air conditioner was not on high enough and I couldn't stay downstairs for dinner. I became so upset and frustrated because I felt that my parents, who best understand my situation, were not paying attention to my needs. My mother became upset because she did not know what more she could do and thought I was overreacting to the temperature, which caused me to become enraged and say a few things that I didn't mean.

In that moment, after all I had been through in the past, I recognized that I wasn't very different; I wasn't much better at controlling my emotions; and that I had in fact changed very little. I also realized that I/we can't make these changes on our own. This is bigger than me/us. We need God in our hearts if we want to change for the better. It's just the reality of the situation.

Be aware of your use of hidden agendas as a method of retrieving information from your partner. Openly state your question or concern. Utilizing hidden agendas to communicate is one of the simplest ways to miscommunicate. For example, during my marriage, from the time I became disabled in 1993 until our divorce, I told my wife on a daily basis what hurt, what was numb, how badly my skin burned, as well as a host of other symptoms. This action would wear on the strongest individual, and it did. My only intention was to let my wife know what symptoms I was experiencing that day, allowing me to track the progress of the disease. In doing this every day in front of her I was hoping that she would realize when I was having an exacerbation and would know that I should see a doctor if that was the case.

I mean, after a while I just couldn't tell when I was getting worse, so I was really just looking for her opinion. In this situation a simple heads-up, an explanation of my purpose for calling attention to my difficulties, pains, and discomforts on a daily basis, could have alleviated a major stressor shouldered by my ex-wife. I never saw the damage I was causing to the relationship until it was too late. Be cognizant of the absolute necessity for clear and open communication between you and your partner.

CHAPTER 5
Worrying about the Future

Y ou may feel that you have been shortchanged, justifiably angry, and miserable, as did I. This is understandable. Disease has dealt a serious blow to your life plans. Planning for one's future and the future of one's family is worrisome enough for the healthiest individual. When worrying becomes overwhelming, there needs to be intervention. I wish I knew then, when I was still married, what I know now.

We all worry, as do many Americans. Worry is "the number one mental health disorder in America" (*Worry-Free Living;* Minirth, Meier, Hawkins, p. 17). Worrying about the future became such a problem for me that it resulted in the loss of my future or, more precisely stated, the future for which I had hoped. In the Bible it says worriers dwell in the "what if's" of life. Live for the day; worrying and stressing will destroy the time you have together with your partner. You must make a conscious team effort to avoid allowing worry and related emotions from taking over your lives.

Worrying as a result of increased vulnerabilities for both you and your family can be very damaging to your relationship if this worry is not properly addressed. Working together with a counselor who is well-educated regarding the difficulties faced by couples dealing with the stresses of life interrupted by a disability or chronic illness is absolutely critical. If you can do this, you and your partner can substantially reduce the stress and stressors in your relationship. One of my biggest regrets is that together my ex-wife and I never sat down and addressed this situation with a counselor specifically trained to assist the disabled and their family members. I'm amazed, and often ask myself how it was that I missed taking this critical step.

Worrying about the future destroys the present and in my case resulted in a future that I could have never imagined. We all have concerns and yes, worries. We just can't let worry overwhelm, dominate or paralyze us. Naturally, we all have concerns about our future and the future of our family members. Every person who takes responsibility seriously can't help but feel a certain amount of worry. Actually, worrying is one reason things get done. There are things like protecting and providing for your loved one(s), life and health insurance, investments, saving for college, all of which become areas of increased concern and vulnerability when your life is interrupted by a disability or chronic illness.

"People who worry are preoccupied or distracted. No matter what else they may be doing, one part of their mind is worrying." ("What Can I Do With My Worry?" Discovery series, p.4). How else could I possibly explain being so oblivious to the hardship and unhappiness suffered for so long by my ex-wife?

In mid-1991 through 1993, my ex-wife and I faced an onslaught of difficulties that would test the strength of our love for one another. First, I changed careers. I had just left a position which I had held for seven years as an analytical chemical technician within the quality assurance laboratory of a powdered infant formula manufacturing company. (What else is one to do with an ecology degree?) Actually, I took that job in 1984 when I realized that working in the outdoors would likely be impossible due to my MS. However, in 1991, I accepted the position of staff scientist/safety coordinator with an environmental testing laboratory. At this time my wife had been working for nine years as an editor for a company that publishes manufacturing textbooks when she was laid off. In an effort to comfort her, I remember jokingly saying, "You know it's summer and you have a six-month severance package. Woo, woo, vacation! I wish I could get laid off like that."

Remember the saying, "Be careful what you wish for"? Well, my wish came true the following week. Little did I know that I would be laid off as well in six months. So we had been engaged to be married for approximately two months, and the two of us, who were comfortable in our careers and previous places of employment, were now out of work. If you are old enough to remember, during the period of the early '90s the economy was not doing very well and corporate America was in the middle of downsizing and just beginning the process of job outsourcing.

Needless to say, the both of us were out of work for quite a while. I did finally get a job as a quality/safety inspector. I, like many people out of work at that time, had no choice but to take a job with a substantial pay cut. After working for a few months, I learned that the company was looking for an administrative assistant. At that time my wife was still pursuing a place of employment. Soon enough, we were both working for the same company. Both my wife and I were earning much less than we had been previously, but finally we were both working again. Our savings account had dwindled to almost nothing. We were barely making enough to meet our mortgage and monthly bills and our credit card balances were growing.

Again, I got laid off. This time, it was April 1993, and the resulting stress had devastating effects. With the disease of multiple sclerosis, increased stress and the worsening of the disease seem to go hand-in-hand. When I became disabled in 1993 just one year after being married, I became overwhelmed with uncertainty and bombarded with questions about the future. How were we going to make it? How would we keep up with the house payments? What were we going to do about health insurance? At thirty-two years of age, practically a newlywed, with an incredible six-year-old stepson, what could I do? What was going to happen to us?

In this situation many people would have become increasingly quiet and withdrawn. That's not my character, but I did have an increase in nervousness, irritability, and anger. Who suffered the consequences? That's right, my innocent and loving wife and stepson. This was a problem that needed professional attention from a counselor who was familiar with working with couples dealing with difficulties and obstacles arising from the introduction of a chronic illness or a disability into the relationship.

Being unemployed and becoming permanently disabled likely placed my ex-wife and me in the most stressful struggle of our lives. Our incomes had been reduced by more than fifty percent over the last two years, and we were about to find ourselves in the middle of yet another battle: The battle to acquire Social Security disability insurance, which turned out to be a process like none I had ever previously experienced.

The process of attaining Social Security disability insurance (SSDI) was truly a battle, which took two extremely stressful years, the help of lawyers, and a letter written by the senator of Vermont to finally win approval. Talk about stress and unnecessary stress at that! It's not that this process was long and tedious; it's more like the many parts of the organization making up the Social Security disability administration seemingly went out of their way to make the process stressful, redundant, and time consuming. I began to feel like the process was specifically designed to wear down even the healthiest of individuals, never mind someone struggling to see, sit in a chair or grasp a writing instrument or eating utensil among other things.

As time went on, it just became blatantly obvious that the disability application process was designed to wear down those that were struggling and in need. By making the applicants jump through hoops and address the same questions with a slightly different slant several times over a period of months and years was beyond frustrating. It was torture. Here's a great example. The first time I was denied SSDI, the reason given was that I had been on disability in the early 1980s, and later in the same decade when the disease went into remission began working again. When the disease worsened during 1993 and I became more severely disabled once again, the Social Security Administration wanted to know why it was that I could work in 1984, but could not work in 1993.

It doesn't take a rocket scientist to understand how this situation could have arisen being that multiple sclerosis is a chronic progressive disease. After reading the questions on the application one could only surmise that the application was being reviewed by a physician with little or no understanding of MS. Thus began the long appeals process, long because I was denied three times and appealed three times. This process consisted of more redundant questions like, how has your condition progressed since your last application? What can't you do today that you could do before? How have things changed that would keep you from working?

Even today my stress level shoots up and my blood begins to boil just thinking about what my ex-wife and I had to deal with. And why? It seems so senseless, unless it was a case of federal bureaucracy designed to encourage the disabled and seniors to give up their quest for federal assistance, which in many cases is a matter of life-and-death. I only hope that this process has been greatly improved over the past fourteen years.

During 1993 my wife and I were also involved in the battle to acquire Betaseron, which at that time was the cutting edge pharmaceutical drug for the treatment of multiple sclerosis. The drug was expensive, costing approximately $980 per month. This was a drug designed to slow or stop the progression of the disease, and we could not afford it. For that reason, I can remember being so upset, depressed, and continually under stress. Imagine having a condition that is progressive for which there is no cure, but now there is a drug treatment that may stop or slow the disease's progression, but the cost prohibits you from using it. It was like being told that it was only to be used to treat the wealthy. I was often so upset and angry that I became confused and frequently could not keep my train of thought. My physical disability and now my cognitive functions had become so limited that I had to rely on my ex-wife to fill out all the endless and maddeningly redundant disability applications.

I can't even begin to tell you how frequently she had to contact their office by phone on my behalf. It wasn't long before my ex-wife and I had figured out that it was seemingly the job of the Social Security disability insurance representatives to wear down, confuse, and discourage us from continuing the process of acquiring Social Security disability insurance. My spirits had become so low. All the stresses and burdens of this process were placed on the back of my ex-wife, and like an over-stuffed backpack it was just another weight added to the cumulative burden of relationship-destroying stress. Before writing this book, I had not realized that after everything my then wife had done for me, I was unable to remember saying thank you. Could that be possible? I was not raised without manners. I loved my ex-wife so very much. I have to believe that I am having a major lapse of memory. If you were raised like me, you would not even think of treating your worst enemy that poorly.

This was the point, June 1993, when I accepted Jesus Christ as my Lord and Savior. After being laid off, my short stint in the hospital, and my resulting permanent disability, I gave in to the request of my friend Chuck, who had asked me several times over the span of several months if I would be interested in attending his church on Sunday. His church, a Bible teaching Pentecostal church, was extremely different, to say the least, in comparison to the teachings of the Catholic church in which I had attended growing up. However, there was something powerfully exhilarating and real about this church service that at first I could not put my finger on. But before too long, I found myself on my knees at the altar giving my then wretched and painfully depressing life to my chosen savior, Jesus Christ. It is not my intention to have this book serve as my testimony for the Lord, but it certainly is not something for which I am ashamed. Just the opposite; miraculous things began to happen in our lives once I accepted Christ, and they were not just by coincidence.

Surprisingly, or more appropriately stated, incredibly, during 1994 we were able to reduce our mortgage and monthly bills by selling our condominium and purchasing a home. We qualified for the home purchase at an extremely low mortgage rate because our household income was so low. However, the week after the closing my ex-wife got a new job with a substantial pay increase and family health benefits that would immediately cover the needs of my pre-existing condition, but that wasn't all. I was also awarded the long-awaited Social Security disability income for which we had been struggling for two years. Had my ex-wife got her new job with the pay increase, or I been awarded disability payments a week earlier, we would not have qualified for our low-rate mortgage. Things were looking up and life was good. A coincidence? I think not!

Of course, the stress of living with the uncertainty of a chronic progressive illness continued to rear its ugly head. To make things worse, the previous owner of the home we purchased in 1995 did not disclose a multitude of serious problems. Since we were down to our last $300 prior to the purchase of our home, we had asked a friend who was a contractor to perform our home inspection. Stop laughing! It was a learning experience. Over the next year and a half, it just happened to be a learning experience with a $40,000 price tag. When the home improvements and repairs were completed, everything had been miraculously paid in full. Thank you, Jesus.

Looking back, I can see that the stress and turmoil of moving into a home that unexpectedly needed so much work— much of which was an immediate safety concern—had me on the edge. It was overwhelming. Within the first two years of owning and living in our first single-family home, we had to face so many issues. For example, we found out the house had serious structural damage resulting from an ongoing problem with carpenter ants that had remained undisclosed by the previous owner. Then we had endless plumbing problems due to the fact that the plumbing was not up to code. The electrical work within the house did not meet safety codes and was a fire hazard. In one case, the previous owner had run new ground wires from the junction box up through the ceiling connected to nothing. (Without a professional home inspection things looked wonderful.) The furnace had been tampered with and was unsafe, so it needed to be replaced. The doors would not close securely, and during the winter months we found out the hard way that all the exterior doors to the house were actually interior doors. The roof and windows leaked profusely. Ultimately, all the exterior doors and windows had to be replaced. The chimney and roof had to be replaced. Beyond that the house was perfect (smile).

I'm sorry to have had to bore you with the problems concerning our residence from 1995 through 1999, but there is a method to my madness. I was hoping to paint a better picture of the physical setting and the emotional state in which my family and I were living during the five-year period from 1995 through May 2000.

I can't stress enough how damaging worrying can be to the body at the cellular level. Remember the saying, "laughter is the best medicine"? There is actually scientific proof of the validity of that statement. The opposite can also be true. Among other things, scientists have found that worriers may be more prone to afflictions such as Alzheimer's, cancer, heart attack, and heart disease.

I want you to see what I missed in hopes of helping you avoid making the same mistakes. I, like millions of others, have a stressful disability that is constantly changing. Every time that I changed careers or went back to school in hopes of retraining for a career more suitable to my level of disability, the level of disability always seemed to change. So staying ahead of the progressive nature of the disease was an ongoing struggle, a game with ever-changing rules and levels of competition.

I think that I can safely assume that because you're reading this book, you, your partner, a family member or friend also deals with a disability or chronic illness that is causing you and yours to be placed in a similarly stressful situation. I hope that by sharing my life experiences with you, they will trigger a light bulb to go on in your head every time you're guilty of making a similar relationship-destroying mistake. You would think that as intelligent human beings we would recognize these situations before the damage was done to our relationships. Obviously, that's not always going to be the case, especially when an unforeseen tragedy, family loss, disability or chronic illness is added to the everyday stresses of one's life.

I snapped one evening in 1996, an episode that I will regret and never forget for the rest of my life. Even now, over a decade later, this incident is painfully difficult for me to discuss. I'm embarrassed and ashamed by my actions and lack of self-control. On that evening my wife and I were arguing, about what, I have no idea. It was probably a situation where we both had just had a bad day and were easily aggravated. As she was walking into the living room and I was passing by her walking out of the living room we were exchanging verbal jabs when I reached out with one arm and pushed her. This was something I had never done before, and never thought of doing. I couldn't imagine raising a hand to my wife. In the heat of the moment it just happened.

The ironic thing was because of my compromised balance and strength, my pushing her caused me to fall over. By the time I got up, she had dialed 911. I asked her to hang up and she did, but as a result of dialing 911 the police were at the house in minutes. Again, no matter what the level of abuse, the abuse cannot be denied. Once you get that label, nobody cares about the level of abuse, you're just given—and rightfully so—the label of domestic abuser.

Just like an episode of "Cops," a patrol car pulled up to the house and two officers came to the front door. Not to make light of the situation, because domestic battery is serious, I have to say the incident that occurred that evening was nothing compared to what you see on the television show. Yet I know that what I did—pushing my spouse—was wrong, appalling, and an action that can never be erased. It was domestic abuse, and I could not deny it happened. Losing my cool in this manner was not like me. For the remainder of my marriage and throughout the divorce process my now ex-wife could and did say to friends, family, and her divorce lawyer that I was abusive, that I had hit or pushed her, and that the police had to come to the house. Even with counseling, the abusive event of that evening would never be forgotten.

When the two police officers arrived, my wife and I were separately interrogated. Our recollection of the incident concurred and the officers agreed not to press charges, partly on the basis of their investigation and partly at the request of my wife. The officers may have been at the house for as long as an hour, but the whole process was surreal and seemingly took hours. Having never been involved with the police for anything other than a traffic ticket, this was a frightening reality check for me. Prior to the officers leaving they requested that I leave for a couple of hours.

After returning home, my wife and I discussed what had happened and how we should proceed. I apologized and swore that nothing like this would ever happen again. Together we planned on making arrangements to seek the help and advice of a social worker who dealt specifically with cases of domestic abuse. The counseling we would receive was absolutely necessary in order to put this event behind us, move forward, and learn how to prevent similar situations from ever occurring again.

I made the mistake of taking care of the physical and forgetting about the emotional. I would make sure I cleaned up after myself in the kitchen, bathroom, anywhere that I created a mess. I would do things like the laundry, help my stepson with his homework, prepare a fresh pot of coffee, or pour two glasses of wine. I performed these small tasks around the house to help make life for my wife less stressful and pleasant. She understood that I did what I could, and she often said that I did more around the house than many husbands that did not even have a disability.

A woman needs to hear how much you love her, why you married her, how beautiful she is, what she means to you as well as how much you really need her. To some degree, a man needs the same support and reassurance. I know that it would certainly have benefited my declining self-esteem and feelings of worthlessness. Remember all the little things like holding hands, a gentle caress, a kiss on the cheek, a sweet gesture of praise. Avoid being critical. Forgetting these things and criticizing your partner will be so damaging to the psyche of your spouse/partner that he or she will likely avoid interacting with you. However, that attention and interaction is needed in the process of supporting and growing the relationship. If you don't provide your partner with this attention, he or she will find it elsewhere.

At work my wife performed at an extremely high level, and she received a lot of recognition and well-deserved praise for that. She was very good, and the resulting recognition and praise that she received on the job was most likely the reason she enjoyed spending more time at work than at home. Where would you rather be, at work receiving recognition and praise or at home receiving criticism from a moody, suffering husband? Well, that's a no-brainer. Please, gather wisdom and knowledge from my mistakes and do everything you can to avoid making the same ones.

I remember my wife telling me that her closest friends and most of the people she interacted with at work were men. One evening, she asked me if I would mind if her friend Tony, a manager from work who lived out-of-state, could come over for dinner. I didn't think that would be a problem. When Tony did come for dinner, the three of us enjoyed a great meal and a couple glasses of wine over conversation. One thing that became obvious to me was my exclusion from ninety percent of the evening's conversation. I first attributed this to the fact that they knew each other quite well from work and it was my first time meeting Tony. When the evening ended and Tony left, I asked Rachel if she had realized that she and Tony excluded me from most of the evening's conversation. She apologized, and I just let it go. But over time, little things like that took a painful toll on my self-esteem. Looking back, I recognize that I never discussed these feelings with my wife. Perhaps if I had engaged my wife in clear and open communication, I would have eliminated my own inner dialogue and aggravation.

I trusted my wife and believed there was nothing going on between her and any other man. I believe that over a long period of not interacting with or paying attention to my wife we just grew apart. My lack of attention was not intentional. It was more a result of the two of us being exhausted. Between my

MS-related fatigue and my wife starting her day at four a.m. we didn't spend much time relating to one another anymore. Many nights she was asleep on the couch by eight thirty. I would awaken her at eleven to go to bed for the evening. By the time I washed up and came to bed she was already asleep. Of course, she didn't want to be awakened, which was understandable because she had to get up in four and a half hours for work. Again, between me being fatigued from MS and her being exhausted from her long days our communication with one another suffered for several years.

CHAPTER 6
Feelings of Inadequacy and Worthlessness

Worthlessness: the big liar. For me the simple tasks and house chores required a lot of effort, but I suppose I felt guilty for not being able to work. Deep down inside, I felt that I had to earn my keep. Accomplishing these tasks, while home alone during the day, gave me a sense of purpose and helpfulness. In paying attention to the physical issues, I unintentionally failed to address the emotional needs of my wife. To make matters worse, I was so physically wiped out, the good that I wanted to do was ironically negated by the fatigue and mean-spiritedness that resulted. All the good things I did during the day were wiped out by the unpleasantness I subjected my dear wife to most nights.

MS-related fatigue and the exhaustive physical struggles changed my mood and personality at the drop of a hat. Over time my moodiness and unintentional mean-spiritedness surely took a toll on my relationship. And another stressor that I was not even aware of at the time was the fact that my wife was watching how difficult, painful, and uncomfortable my life had become. Many times that fact alone can be enough to make the strongest individual want to escape the situation.

Neurologists recognize that the symptoms of MS worsen during the middle to later part of the day. This differs for everyone, but I noticed and struggled from the worsened symptoms, especially MS-related fatigue between the hours of three o'clock in the afternoon until about ten o'clock at night.

Unless you are familiar with MS or suffer from the disease yourself, you probably don't understand the extent of the symptoms of the disease. For a healthy individual, fatigue might be a feeling of sleepiness or a feeling of complete exhaustion. But anyone who is familiar with MS-related fatigue knows that those three words describe a condition way beyond exhaustion. Physically, MS-related fatigue feels more like one's arms, legs or torso are filled with concrete. Your mind tells your body to lift your leg but nothing happens. You may begin to bend at the knees or waist, but the body uncontrollably continues to collapse in on itself like a building imploding during a scheduled demolition.

My wife usually walked in from work around six o'clock when I was suffering at my worst. The appropriate reaction to seeing one's spouse after a long day should certainly be a happy greeting, a warm hug, a kiss, a loving caress, but nine out of ten times that wasn't the case. More often than not, just to get onto my feet at that time of day was impossible. I did my best to share a kiss and if energy allowed a brief hug, more often than not from a sitting or lying position. Movements were difficult. I was weak, and I took the frustration and anger arising from feelings of inadequacy, guilt, uselessness, and embarrassment of the obvious physical struggle to function, out on my wife. And the worst thing was I allowed this scenario to persist night after night.

As a man, I know I felt like a failure. After all, men are supposed to be the providers, right? At my church, I facilitated a course entitled "Life Interrupted" where participants learned that the healthy partner/caregiver is powerful and the disabled partner is especially sensitive to being spoken down to, belittled, and disrespected. Being disrespected often results in anger, silence, and feelings of inadequacy felt by the disabled partner, which frequently leads to that partner openly expressing anger or just withdrawing completely from any type of interaction or problem resolution. Without resolution, the bitter feelings, anger, and disappointment are just put away and continue to build internally until a later date. Inevitably, the internal pressure builds to the point where all the pressure explodes like a volcano expressing itself as an uncontrolled eruption of anger and hostility.

Feelings of worthlessness are more destructive to a relationship than one recognizes. Anger is a response to the loss of self-worth. I felt that my ex-wife thought I was becoming worthless as I became more disabled. You're probably thinking, Chris, you were assuming the feelings that someone else may or may not have been experiencing. If so, you would be correct and much of the time my assumption was incorrect. In making this blind assumption one only increases one's own feelings of worthlessness.

But for me, this was not a completely blind assumption. This statement arose from a conversation my ex-wife and I had in which I expressed my concern for her safety while being in the house alone. I think that I was going away for the weekend when I brought up the subject. Her response was "if something were to happen what could you do anyway?" I'm sure that she did not mean for her statement to be so hurtful, but as the man of the house it had just that effect, because it made me feel worthless.

This reminds me of the lyrics to an old Eagles song which states, "We often live our lives in chains not even knowing we hold the key." When an individual is disrespected or made to feel worthless, whether he or she is disabled or not, that person often becomes angry and defensive. I know I was often responsible for reacting to that situation in this manner.

Again, not to make an excuse, but because the symptoms of MS worsen during the hours of three and ten p.m. (the approximate times may differ) as a result of physical activities and/or environmental factors like temperature and humidity, when my wife arrived home from work around six o'clock, I was usually miserable and struggling to function. One needs to make a conscious effort to minimize projecting one's misery and resulting anger onto those who mean the most to you. If you continue to let this happen, like me, one day you could hear your spouse/partner say, "I feel numb, and I don't know if I love you anymore." And most likely, you, like me, will have no idea how this happened.

I'll never forget hearing those words on October 27, 2000. My then wife was sitting on the couch watching a Red Sox ballgame. I had just gotten up to get something from the other room when I asked her an innocent question, which surprisingly drew an irritated response. I said to her, "Is something wrong? Lately, you seem to be irritated with me."

She replied by stating, "I feel numb, and I don't know if I love you anymore." I remember responding by jokingly asking, "So what do you want, a *divorce*?" I was shocked when she said that she didn't know and that she thought I should leave for a while.

To put it lightly, this didn't go over well with me. Her thinking was that if I left for a while she would see if she missed me, which would let her know that she still loved me. I couldn't believe what I was hearing. She suggested that I should go stay with my mother down in Massachusetts.

My first thought was: "Wouldn't it be easier for you, the healthy partner, to move out for a while?" After all, I was comfortable functioning in our house because of the open floor plan, handicapped accessibility, and familiarity with the overall contents of the home. Her thinking was that if I went to my mother's down in Massachusetts, my mother would make my life easier by caring for me. I ended up spending about a month back home, during which time I saw a counselor while my wife also received counseling up in Vermont.

I received a phone call on November 27 from my wife. She said that she loved me and that she wanted me to come home. I swear that was the happiest moment of my life. I thought everything was going to work out. I was so excited that I took a flight from Boston's Logan Airport to Burlington International Airport in Vermont the next morning. I couldn't get back to my family fast enough. I felt like I had just received a pardon from the governor from a death sentence. I had a future again; what an incredible wave of emotion. Words couldn't possibly express the happiness I felt knowing that my wife still loved me.

Personal notes, thoughts and memories, concepts and Ideas, that I would like to put into practice:

After returning home on the 28th of November, my wife and I decided that we should continue counseling as a couple after the first of the year. We decided to treat the month of December like everything was fine and that there had never been a problem, all the time knowing that after the first of the year we were going to seek marriage counseling. I thought the intention was to rectify any unresolved issues as well as learn how to better handle the stress and difficult times that we could face. There is a lot to absorb, face, and handle when husband and wife become patient and caregiver.

Overall, December turned out to be a great month. Prior to the beginning of the month, my wife and I had a discussion at which time she made it clear that I should not expect her to say that she loved me when I said I loved her, because, as she put it, "she wasn't there yet."

I understood that, or at least I thought I did. I interpreted that as I should not be saying I love you or giving her praise because it would make her feel uncomfortable because she was unable to return those feelings at that time. To quote another country song, I'd say that we had an "I'm gonna hate myself in the morning, but I'm gonna love you tonight" kind of relationship.

Looking back, that month-long relationship was likely the reason that the discussion during our first counseling session in January came as such a shock to me. I thought things were pretty good between my wife and me. I was just waiting for the okay from my wife—the okay that would let me know it was all right to express and show my loving and caring emotions. Remember, I was thinking that I was not supposed to be sharing these feelings with my wife until she was able to return those feelings.

CHAPTER 7
Counseling: what you should know

The counselor started by asking my wife the following two-part question: How do you think things are going and what are you feeling? She responded by saying that because she was there she must want the relationship to work. Then she dropped the bomb. She said that she didn't love me. I had no idea that she felt that way. She had said that she loved me when she wanted me to come home to Vermont in November. We had a great Christmas together. There were few if any disagreements during the month, yet she said that she didn't love me.

I was devastated. How could that be? I needed an explanation and my wife couldn't provide one. Remember the elation, the high that came over me after the phone call from my wife in November when she said that she loved me and wanted me to come home? As high as that moment had been, this moment was equally as low. I felt as though I had just been punched in the stomach and couldn't catch my breath.

I was surprised when the counselor had nothing to say, no guidance or input whatsoever. We met with this counselor for two more sessions, still with no guidance or input before she suggested that we see separate counselors. The counselor didn't say it, but the reason she suggested that we see separate counselors was pretty obvious. During the three sessions with this particular counselor, communication between my wife and me had begun to break down and become more adversarial in the presence of the counselor. That was more than fine with me, because the counselor whom Rachel and I had been seeing provided us with nothing. Just from what I knew about a therapist's occupation, which was little more than what I had seen on the television and in the movies, I knew that she should have been actively listening to what we, as individuals and as a couple, had to say. Actively listening involves paraphrasing, validating, and affirming your partner's input/feelings. I was under the impression that the desired goal was to carry on with our separate counselors to determine if we should again meet as a couple with another counselor, a counselor who was familiar with the marital issues, concerns, and trials facing a couple whose lives had been complicated by the introduction of chronic illness or disability. I was not prepared to drop the issue or give up after coming this far.

So my wife and I scheduled appointments to meet separately with separate psychologists. I had seen my psychologist for three sessions before my wife was scheduled to meet with hers. She came in one evening after she was supposed to have had her first meeting with the psychologist. I asked her how it went, and she responded that she had not gone to her appointment. She said that she had met with a lawyer that afternoon and that she wanted a divorce. In preparation for the divorce process I got a lawyer, and things spiraled downhill from there. Our divorce was finalized on December 1, 2001.

As a disabled individual or the caregiver at the end of a bad day, when we are struggling or when we are feeling at our worst both mentally and physically, our spouses or partners— the ones whom we most love and care about—bear the brunt of our struggles, pain, and frustration. And because they love us so much, know our innermost feelings, and understand better than anyone else what we are going through, despite our bearishness they put up with us for as long as they can. However, a marital counselor who deals with the stresses that are introduced into a relationship as a result of a chronic illness or disability can be extremely helpful within the process of saving your relationship.

If you allow the "Poor Me Attitude" to persist like I did, you may find that no matter what you do or say, it will upset your spouse. You will have become an irritant no matter what you do. For example, you might become upset or laugh when you fall, and it's the wrong way to react in the eyes of your once loving and caring spouse. I know this because for years if I tripped and fell or spilled a cup of coffee my reaction was one of anger. Even if this anger was not directed at my wife, my undirected misery and anger certainly made her feel sad and uncomfortable.

I later learned to find humor and laugh at myself rather than react with misplaced anger. This reaction also became upsetting. Soon I realized that it did not matter how I reacted. I remember one evening my wife and I were entertaining our neighbors, a Christian couple with whom we had developed a very close relationship, when I tripped and fell over my walker. Like most MS-related falls, spills or unexplained mishaps, they seem to happen so quickly and without a cause. I have chalked this phenomenon up to not taking the necessary time and thought to safely negotiate what now goes into making what was once one's simple next move.

Nevertheless, I reacted by laughing and making light of the situation. We all seemed to enjoy a good laugh once the others noticed that I had not gotten hurt. Later that evening, after our friends had gone, to my surprise my wife expressed her disapproval over how I had handled the situation. I remember she said, "You know, they could see right through your laughter." I don't know if she felt that I had overcompensated for my embarrassment by seeing humor in what could have been an uncomfortable situation had the couple not been such close friends. What I did know was that at this point in our marriage no matter how I reacted, it was irritating and wrong in the eyes of my wife.

In another situation, putting or not putting my arm around my wife was a problem. If I didn't put my arm around my wife, I was guilty of not showing that I cared; however, when I did put my arm around her, because my arm felt too heavy because of limited sensation, that was a problem.

This was the point at which I realized no matter what my reaction, it was going to be wrong. I had seemingly become nothing more than an irritant. One cannot improve a situation like this if you believe there is no answer. Saying there is no answer is like giving up and giving in. I did not realize that that was exactly what I was doing. I should have explained to my wife why my arm felt so heavy when I put it around her at night. Instead, rather than putting my arm around her, I just lay in bed next to her, night after night. She may have misinterpreted my behavior as a lack of compassion or interest in our relationship.

Early on in my marriage I remember saying to my wife, "If the shoe were on the other foot and you had multiple sclerosis, I don't know if I could deal with the emotional heartbreak and stress." She responded by saying that I would never become a burden and that she had known what she could be getting into before we got married. However, neither she nor I had counted on the emotional burden which we eventually had to confront. In retrospect, I don't think anyone faced with the situation for the first time would be able to handle the situation without counseling.

I know a couple dealing with marital stress brought on by the misfortune of an unexpected disability. As with my situation, Sandy, the wife, is in the role of the caregiver and she's struggling emotionally. At one point she shared with me how she just wanted to be treated like a wife and not a caregiver. When I heard Sandy say this, I knew and understood for the first time exactly the feelings with which my ex-wife had been dealing. This revelation was like I had just walked into a brick wall and the collision knocked the cobwebs from my brain. I'm sure my ex-wife felt the same way. I'm sure Sandy, as well as my ex-wife and most people for that matter, did not and do not have a problem with providing their spouse with assisted care and filling the role of caregiver. The situation becomes an issue when the individual in the role of the caregiver is no longer shown love, compassion, appreciation, and respect.

Remember to tell your partner frequently that you love her/him, let her/him know that you cherish her/him, hug her/him, hold her/his hand. I was suffering from the fatigue and other symptoms of multiple sclerosis, and what I didn't do, I needed to do and you must do. You have to show your love and appreciation for everything that your spouse/partner does for you. As couples, we need to stay in touch with the special ways of growing, refreshing, and rejuvenating our relationships. It may be more difficult because of your present situation, illness or disability, but what's the alternative? Don't forget or give up on that which first drew you to one another like a moth to a flame or a fly to...well, a moth to the flame (smile).

Don't allow the counselor to "make it all about you." I suggest that you and your spouse seek a counselor, particularly one who deals with those struggling with a disability or chronic progressive illness such as MS, ALS, cerebral palsy or Alzheimer's and the like. When an individual or couple sees a counselor for anything, marital advice, depression, domestic abuse, alcohol or drug abuse, anything, just be aware of biased advice. I say biased because many times a counselor may unintentionally tilt the table by providing suggestions designed to make life easier for the disabled partner, forgetting to address the needs of the caregiver altogether. I recall my ex-wife and me seeing several counselors as a couple and because my disability was obvious because of my wheelchair the counselor frequently addressed issues that would improve or make life easier for me. At this time I had been taking the antidepressant Zoloft for my depression. Why had an antidepressant only been prescribed for me? After seeing and hearing about all the difficulties that my ex-wife was going through, wouldn't you think that the counselor would have prescribed an antidepressant for my wife as well? The well spouse/caregiver, also needs care, compassion, and advice. The counselor should be there to help both of you. After all, the couple is suffering from the disability or illness. "It's not all about me." It's really about improving life for *us.*

My wife and I once had an experience with a counselor who made suggestions designed to reduce stress on me by getting me out of the house and into the neighborhood with my wheelchair. Not one time did the counselor refer to how we as a couple could work together to reduce stress for each other. How about reducing the stress on us? Apparently, even the counselor thought "It Was All About Me." I know that my wife felt invisible and alone. Alone, because a professional whose job it was to help us identify and deal with a difficult situation did not even recognize that I was not the only one struggling, depressed, and at the end of my rope. In time, I found out that my wife took this very hard. Who can blame her? After that session, she did not know where to turn. When I think about this, how alone and trapped she must have felt, I want to cry.

I put my ex-wife on a pedestal because I thought that she was so great and so understanding, but I never thought to get her help or support. In my weakness, I thought she was so strong, a mortal wonder-woman, but everyone in her situation needs physical, medical or psychological help at some point. Of course, the risk of putting someone on top of a pedestal is that you are placing that individual in a precarious and dangerous position. My ex-wife hated it when I put her on a pedestal because inevitably, like all of us, she would make a mistake and I would let her know it. She could never understand how I, the person who loved her, could turn in anger and knock her down from the position of praise. At that time, I did not recognize the hurtful and irreversible damage for which I was responsible.

There will be days in everyone's marriage when, in anger or frustration, you or your spouse will react to a situation in a way that is out of control and inappropriate. Rather than cutting one another down, being argumentative or adding fuel to the fire, instead become aware of the situation and put a stop to it immediately. Allowing a heated argument like this to continue guarantees the likelihood that something will be said that cannot be taken back. Instead, remember why you fell in love in the first place. Was it humor, truthfulness, passion, chemistry, wisdom, success or patience? Whatever it was remember that person, the person you're about to hurt with words and actions that you can never take back.

We can and should always apologize and ask our partner for forgiveness. Because hurtful and hate-filled behavior from one's partner is never totally forgotten, this behavior must be eliminated from your life. It's not acceptable behavior by anyone, especially a married couple. Now, we all know that disagreements and arguments are inevitable. They are a natural part of every relationship. However, they must not be allowed to become an emotional, venomous, hate-filled bashing of one another.

In our marriages and closest relationships there will be plenty of opportunity to notice one another's flaws. There will be times where we have to hold one another to account or suggest a change and that can be difficult. Of course, many of us know from experience that our spouses or partners may not respond well to such a suggestion.

So how can we navigate these waters? To avoid the situation would be irresponsible and destructive to one's marriage in the long run. Incorrectly, rather than face this touchy or confrontational situation I chose to avoid it altogether. The problem with this behavior is that all of the unresolved issues build up until the inevitable explosion of pent-up frustration. This point in the conversation, if you can call it that, is anything but rational and beneficial to one's relationship.

At this point the responsible approach would be to ask your partner for forgiveness if you have contributed to the problem. Generally this is a question that doesn't need to be asked because most if not all confrontations are the result of contributions by both parties. Forgiveness and caring communication, rather than silence or hurtful criticism, is needed.

Never avoid addressing the problem. It is important to ensure that there has been an acceptable resolution to the problem prior to putting the matter to rest. Never assume, like most guys do, that because the fighting has subsided or your partner has become quiet that everything has been forgotten and things are fine. I can guarantee with 99.9 percent certainty that the problem will surely arise again when it's least expected if the problem has not been resolved. The next time you're feeling a little frisky and you're in the mood, you will surely find out that things have not been forgotten. Sure, you may be smiling now, but I suggest you heed my warning.

CHAPTER 8
Final Thoughts and Personal Regrets

In the end, do you know what hurt the most? I believe that in ninety-five percent of all divorces in America today, what hurts the most is no surprise. It's the tearing, ripping, and extrication of part of one's self when the couple is torn apart, resulting in two emotionally wounded individuals. A simple analogy, one which probably most clearly describes that which has just taken place, can best be described by looking at a piece of rope. Think of a piece of rope as two separate strands intertwined to create one strong, solid rope. As in a marriage or relationship two separate individuals, like two separate strands of rope, intertwine to become one. When the couple is ripped apart by divorce like the ripping apart of the strands that make up the rope, parts of the couple are torn from one another. It can be very emotional when intimate parts of oneself are removed as the result of a couple splitting. These losses make a divorce agonizing and difficult to get over. It's these gaping holes that leave the individuals vulnerable to the sometimes painful mistake known as the so-called rebound relationship. This is why divorce is so painful and in many cases may take years to work through and get over. For obvious reasons the length of time it takes to get over a divorce is often proportional to the length of the relationship or marriage.

The second cause of pain or hurt, and in my case the most hurtful and devastating loss, was the stealing away of the great memories that once were. I mean, whenever a couple breaks up or divorces, they can look into one another's eyes and ask what happened, how did we lose our love, when did this happen or where did we go wrong? No matter how you phrase the question, at least the question and the emotions are there. This is the point where as a couple you may share your final tearful and caring embrace. Isn't it ironic that this almost loving moment is the result of the impending divorce? You both know that it's over, but you look into one another's hearts via those beautiful eyes (in my case my ex-wife's beautiful big blue eyes) and realize what was once awesome is gone.

I was devastated by one hurtful statement from my ex-wife that was delivered with the same shocking pain experienced by a single misplaced hammer blow to the thumb. I will never forget it. My ex-wife and I were big fans of country music and we really enjoyed a song by Garth Brooks entitled "The Dance." Within the lyrics of the song Mr. Brooks sings:

"Looking back on the memory of the dance we shared for a moment all the world was right,

how could I have known that you'd ever say goodbye and now I'm glad I didn't know the way it all would end, the way it all would go.

Our lives are better left to chance, I could've missed the pain but I'd a had to miss the dance..."

I remember my ex-wife saying, "I wish I had missed the dance." That cut like a knife. I just thought of all the wonderful times, incredible moments, experiences, and laughs only to wonder how that statement could have ever come from her mouth. After all, we had shared so many tremendous experiences, like our annual stays on Martha's Vineyard, trips to Lake Placid, New York, and vacationing in the Dominican Republic, just to name a few. Plus, we enjoyed similar passions together like designing, planting, and caring for our extravagant perennial gardens, watching sports and movies, or trying and sharing a new wine.

After a hard day's work, many evenings we would sit down at the coffee table or out on the deck with a nice bottle of red wine and talk while sharing cheese a crackers, Greek olives or just a bag of chips. I loved those times and cherished those moments spent together. I'll never forget them. They will just fade away over time like a great day concludes with the sun setting into the sea or behind the trees.

Yes, divorce brings out the worst, but there should be no denying the loving, caring, giving, and joyful times, referred to as "The Dance," that existed earlier in the marriage. In the case of my divorce, I pray that this kind of hate will dissipate over time. Bitterness, like a cancer, left alone to grow only destroys one's life no matter what the cause. Whether it is sparked by a hateful divorce that is the result of the misery of a chronic illness, the tragic loss of a loved one or any other tragic interruption to one's life, a certain level of forgiveness and coming to terms with one's past has to take place. Without this coming to terms and letting go of the past which has caused you so much pain, one's life will be consumed by the bitterness. Moving on requires forgetting, forgiving, and loving others like you love yourself so that you are free to find happiness again. Life goes on and true happiness is out there. I'm living proof.

My hope is that you will have learned and benefited from me sharing my personal experiences, mistakes, and failures.

Again, if just one relationship is saved or benefited from reading this book, the sharing of my personal story and the putting into words of my heartfelt thoughts will have been well worth it.

I truly believe that if I had taken five minutes a day to sit down on the couch with my wife, put my arm around her, rest her head on my shoulder and ask her, "Honey, how are you doing?" then really taking the time to listen to what she had to say would have gone a long way in the process of not only saving but growing my relationship. Your spouse/partner needs to be able to see how caring, compassionate, and literally invested in her/him and your relationship you are. And this shouldn't be a difficult task. After all, you love this person with your whole heart, and he or she deserves to know how much you love and respect him or her. You would do anything for this individual, but because of your physical hardships you, like me, may be unable. This does not give us the right to ignore the feelings of others. It's sad, but many times we forget these simple loving truths in our lives and we need to go out of our way to refocus on these the most important truths in our lives.

If there is one thing that I have learned from all this, it is that we would be best served if we were able to say and react to things in slow motion. If we could learn to think of what we were going to say and how it was going to sound before the words were to ever leave our mouths, and likewise think of how we were going to react to something and what that was going to look or sound like, maybe we could consciously avoid hurting one another. Because our hardships create such frustration, anger and anxiety we lose sight of how hurtful and unacceptable we are acting.

As important as it is to have and demonstrate compassion, it is just as important to avoid acting with a lack of compassion.

It doesn't matter how much compassion you demonstrate one minute if you demonstrate an equal or greater lack of compassion the next. For example, there was one point in our lives, before I knew how much a human could love a dog, that I demonstrated a major lack of compassion. My wife and I had just gotten married when her dog was hit and killed by an automobile. When we went to bed that evening she began to cry over the loss of her dog. Never having had a dog myself, I said, "Why are you crying? It was only a dog." At that time, all I could think of was that I had to get up at six a.m. Sleep was so very important to me. The symptoms of multiple sclerosis would flare up when I received less than eight hours of sleep. All I was thinking about was me.

Again we need to slow things down. If you were to take a second to think about who's the most important person in the world, and many times we don't, you would recognize the need to show your love and compassion for your partner not only in his/her time of need, but always. I should have, and you should let your partner know that when he or she needs comfort your loss of sleep is not an issue. I wish I had done that. Expressing that bit of compassion over the years would surely have had a positive cumulative effect. Alone, this would not likely have changed the outcome of my marriage, but in addition to all the other changes and adjustments, I think we would have made it. Save the battles for the big issues—and you'll have a happy relationship.

I don't know if your relationship is or was like mine, but I can remember when my marriage first began and my then wife and I had very little money, few possessions, and as I would soon learn, very few concerns, worries, and a limited amount of stress compared to what everyday family life would inevitably bring down the pike. All too often we find out too late that we had it all when all we had was each other.

In my prayers, I pray that I can live all that I have learned. By the grace of God, my new fiancee, Jane, and I plan to be married in the spring of 2007.

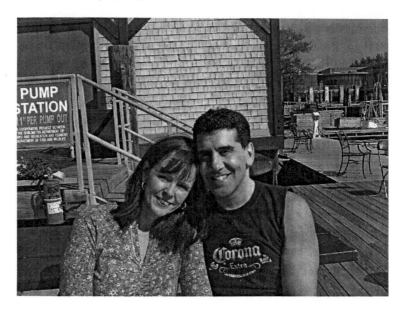

Jane and I, visiting the Burlington waterfront in late August 2006, after visiting with my stepson Jesse who is now himself twenty and attending college in Vermont.

We have purchased a beautiful home in Holliston, just forty feet from my parents who live next door in the house where I was raised. It will be quite surreal and funny in many ways, because as a child some of my best friends lived in the home in which I now live. I played hide and go seek and I ran around playing soccer in this very same backyard and, as a teenager, in the '70s, I spent many days swimming in the very same pool that I now own.

I love the layout of our new house. The house, a colonial, has been renovated so that the entire first floor of the house is now completely accessible to me utilizing a wheelchair or walker. On the first floor, the dining room and one bay of the two-car garage have been converted into our master bedroom suite with a handicapped accessible master bath. The backyard, patio, and pool are all on the same level providing for easy accessibility from our oversized great room, which looks out onto the pool. The in-ground swimming pool will surely provide many afternoons of fun and entertainment. Having the pool will allow me to participate in outdoor activities and enjoy the heat of the summer once again. For years I have dreaded the approaching summer season, because of how the heat negatively affects my MS. Access to a pool, our pool, will change that.

I am so looking forward to spending this summer and every summer to come with my new family. Jane is so beautiful, caring, and full of compassion and life. She is a dream come true, and truly an answer to my prayers. Jane has three children, Michael, 23, Lauren, 20, and Mark, 16, all of whom are impressive, intelligent young adults whose lives I look forward to sharing and being a part.

Closing Prayer:

Please, Lord, destroy my foolish pride, guide me down paths of good sense and smart choices, and keep my mouth from hurting anyone, especially those dearest to me. Purify my thoughts and direct my words so that when I speak, the words that flow from my mouth reflect Your grace and love.

There can be no answer apart from You. You, Heavenly Father, are aware of and in control of all situations, good and bad. Please guide me and provide me with Your strength and hope. See me through everything that I do.

Father, help me by the power of Your Spirit to truly love my partner, always. Help me to think not only of my life but also the life of my partner and all God's people. Having received the gift of God's love, may I pass this love on to those I love. I pray this in Christ's most holy name, Amen.

THE END

APPENDIX A
The Miracles of Bee Venom Therapy (BVT)

This appendix has been added to the book not because it has anything to do with the stresses added to a relationship because of the introduction of a chronic illness or disability, but rather as a source of information that may add some relief to those who suffer from inflammatory diseases such as multiple sclerosis and arthritis.

In this appendix you will be introduced to a form of alternative medicine that involves being stung by honeybees with the desired result of reducing inflammation, thus ultimately reducing the symptoms of my MS. The symptoms of inflammatory diseases like arthritis and multiple sclerosis worsen with increased inflammation. Remember that within the disease process of multiple sclerosis, the myelin (the protective sheath) covering the spinal cord and nerves— basically the entire central nervous system—is damaged, reducing neurological function directly related to the swelling of the scars. If you are interested in learning more about Bee Venom Therapy, I recommend reading the book *How Well Are You Willing to Bee* by Pat Wagner. You can also visit her web site beelady@olg.com or by conducting a search on "the bee lady." Pat Wagner, known as "the Bee Lady," has had multiple sclerosis for more than twenty-five years, and in her book she shares the story of her miraculous healing. Because of Pat Wagner's positive experiences with bee sting therapy (apitherapy), I thought I would give the honeybees a try.

Although my improvements are a mere shadow of those experienced by Pat Wagner, to me they have been mind-blowing. If I hadn't experienced them myself, I would be more than a little skeptical, which by the way is exactly what I had been for twenty-plus years regarding the treatment of multiple sclerosis with bee stings. At the present time, I have been stung approximately 11,000 times over the past three years. I'm not in love with the pain inflicted by my little buzzing buddies; however, the results are frequently so great the pain is nothing more than a mere nuisance.

I began the process of Bee Venom Therapy (BVT) on July 5, 2003, thanks to my dear friend Brenda and her girls, Brittany and Rebecca, with some pretty incredible results, some of which I would like to share with you. I'm not a doctor, and I am not suggesting that you try BVT. I just want to share my results with you and let you know that BVT is being used as an alternative treatment for multiple sclerosis and other inflammatory disorders. If you are considering using the honeybee as an alternative method of treatment because of the information I am sharing, you should first consult your own physician. The information herein should not be construed as the practice of medicine. The following are results that I have experienced while undergoing what is commonly known as Bee Venom Therapy.

Results I have experienced:

07/11/03: Seven stings, 6 on lower back, 1 on right outer ankle;
Almost immediately my right foot, which was blue and cold, became warm with a normal to pinkish skin tone.

07/12/03: Increased movement of my right foot up, down, and side to side, after having limited movement of that foot since 1993. Almost immediately I had color and warmth in my foot where moments before it was blue and ice cold.

07/13/03: I experienced increased energy and stamina. I was able to stand and support myself with just one hand on the back of a chair while I danced at church...hallelujah!!

I was able to stand up with perfect posture and keep my balance unassisted; for the first time in five years my back was no longer hunched over. It was no longer difficult to hold up my torso (these improvements lessened over the next two to three hours).

07/23/03: Fourteen stings, 2 on shoulder blades, 10 on the back/spine.

07/24/03: Today, I have increased strength and energy. As usual, I worked out on my Total Gym. Today, however, I was able to work out midday, which is usually impossible as I usually have no energy at that time of day.

08/05/03: Twenty stings, all 20 on my back; For the third time, stinging my back has provided me with the ability to stand up straight, keep my balance, and function more easily. For about a month now, I have been able to shower standing up whereas before I started bee venom therapy I was using a seat in the shower. Maybe more information than you need to know, smile.

08/07/03: I was able to have a great workout on my Total Gym. As in the past, when I have experienced functional improvement the day after being stung, the improvements are limited to increased energy and stamina. The other improvements, such as reduced spasticity/tone, improved balance, and the ability to stand up straight have not lasted through the night.

10/05/03: Thirty stings, 20 on legs, 2 on knees, 2 on ankles, 6 on arms; I was immediately able to stand straight, and I walked using minimal support on the walker. I was able to walk onto and across the deck, turn around, and walk back across the deck into the house without the walker or any outside assistance (approximately twenty-five steps). I was able to walk upstairs easily (fourteen stairs). I then had a tremendous workout on the Total Gym with a higher than usual level of energy.

This was by far the greatest improvement I have had to this point after starting BVT on July 5, 2003.

02/07/04: Thirty three stings, nineteen on legs, four on hips, four on ankles, six on knees; Immediately able to stand up straight, noticeably improved balance, stability, energy, and emotional improvement.

03/08/04: Twenty-two stings, ten on kidneys, four on feet, eight on ankles; Immediately I was able to stand up straight and walk around the kitchen without a walker (using the counter for support), increased energy, strength, and stamina. The stings eliminated the spasticity/tone that just moments before was keeping me from being able to bend and move my legs. Movements became effortless, plus I had greatly improved balance.

03/14/04: Twenty-four stings, eight on legs, four on knees, eight on hands, four on arms; Prior to being stung I could not get off the floor or move my arms or legs, then immediately after being stung I was able to stand up straight and move my arms and legs. My energy level, strength, and stamina were through the roof. I was able to work out three times during the next six hours, amazing!

04/17/05: Twenty-two stings, six on legs, two on Achilles tendon, ten on kidneys, four on lower back;
I was able to go up fourteen stairs taking only seven simple steps. Prior to those twenty-two stings, I was using a chair lift because I was unable to lift my legs. Absolutely incredible!

05/01/05: Twenty-two stings, four on lower back, ten on kidneys, eight on legs;

Prior to getting stung, I was hunched over, struggling to walk with my walker because my legs were so stiff with spasticity/tone, but after being stung I was able to stand up straight and walk using my walker. The spasticity and tone were eliminated, allowing me to stand and move with improved balance and fluidity. At church I was able to stand worshiping God in song and fellowship with friends (holding the back of a chair).

3/05/06: Twenty-two, two on wrists, six on hands, eight on knees, six on feet/ankles.

3/06/06: Yesterdays good results were short-lived, but the following day was an extremely good day with high energy and the increased ability to function, most noticeably the ability to walk more easily using my walker.

(Total stings as of January 16, 2007 was 12,310)

That is just a sampling of the changes and results that I've seen since I began BVT in July 2003. I had an MRI scan of my brain conducted in 2003 prior to beginning the bee stinging process and again in 2004. The MRI scan has shown no significant increase of lesions on my brain. Doctors do not seem to want to acknowledge that the use of BVT has resulted in improved motor function or slowing the process of disease progression. At times, I am tempted to believe that this reaction could have been predicted. You hear so many individuals stating that the treatment of disease using natural and holistic methods is not profitable for the big pharmaceutical companies, resulting in little or no research involving these forms of possible remedies. I happen to be a proponent of disease treatment utilizing both the pharmaceutical and holistic approaches to medicine.

APPENDIX B

The ABC's of Pharmaceutical Disease Management for the Treatment of Multiple Sclerosis

Over the years, I have been treated with each of the so-called ABC drugs (Avonex, Betaseron and Copaxone). All of which have proven in clinical trials to be effective treatments for relapsing-remitting forms of multiple sclerosis. From my experience with these treatments, I can tell you that it is extremely difficult to determine how much these drug protocols aid in the process of disease management. For example, at times I felt like the disease was progressing faster while taking the medication. It is very difficult to determine if the disease is progressing more quickly or more slowly than it would have had I not been taking the medication. Frequent MRI scans of the brain are the best way to identify active disease. Several times I stopped taking a medication because I felt like I was progressing more rapidly while on the drug. However, there wais no way to determine if this was a result of the drug treatment or just the natural course of the disease. You'll have to draw your own conclusions, but most physicians recommend being on one of the following drugs as a necessary part of the management of multiple sclerosis.

Avonex is produced by and a registered trademark of Berlex Pharmaceuticals. Avonex is approved by the FDA to treat relapsing forms of multiple sclerosis to decrease the number of flare-ups and slow the occurrence of some of the physical disability that is common with individuals who suffer from MS. I underwent the once a week treatment with Avonex from late 1997 through mid 2000. If you would like to find out more about the treatment with Avonex call 1-800-456-2255

Betseron produced by and a registered trademark of Biogen- Idec. Betaseron is a highly effective treatment for multiple sclerosis, which has been shown to keep 73 percent more patients relapsed free with Betaseron versus placebo at one year. Talk to your doctor or contact a BETA nurse at 1-800-877-1467

Copaxone is produced by and a registered trademark of Teva Pharmaceutical Industries. Copaxone is indicated for the reduction of relapses in relapsing remitting multiple sclerosis as well as the reduction of new brain lesions. At the present time I am receiving treatment daily with Copaxone. If you would like to find out more about treatment with Copaxone, please call shared solutions at 1-800-887-8100.

Personal notes, thoughts and memories, concepts and Ideas, that I would like to put into practice: